The Chinese Hospital

The Chinese Hospital

A Socialist Work Unit

GAIL E. HENDERSON AND
MYRON S. COHEN

YALE UNIVERSITY PRESS
NEW HAVEN and LONDON

Published with assistance from the foundation established
in memory of Amasa Stone Mather of the class of 1907,
Yale College.

Designed by James J. Johnson
and set in Galliard Roman type by Eastern Graphics.
Printed in the United States of America by
Edwards Brothers, Inc., Ann Arbor, Michigan.

Library of Congress Cataloging in Publication Data

Henderson, Gail, 1949–
    The Chinese hospital.

    Bibliography: p.
    Includes index.
    1. Hospitals—China—Sociological aspects.
2. Hu-pei sheng i hsueh yüan. Fu shu ti 2 i yüan.
I. Cohen, Myron, S.   II. Title.   III. Title: Danwei.
RA990.C5H46   1984   362.1′1′095121   83-16943
ISBN 0–300–03063–0

*The paper in this book meets the guidelines for
permanence and durability of the Committee on Production
Guidelines for Book Longevity of the Council on Library
Resources.*

10 9 8 7 6 5 4 3 2 1

To our daughter, Jessie,
a world traveler at an early age

Contents

Illustrations follow pages 26, 65, and 109.

List of Figures and Tables

Preface

In the years since the Cultural Revolution (1966–1976), an increasing number of Western journalists and scholars have had the opportunity to live in the People's Republic of China for prolonged periods. The result has been a flow of books that provides a more realistic perception of China's complexity. Nevertheless, in a manner reminiscent of the old imperial style, the leaders of the Communist regime have welcomed only limited contact with Westerners. For journalists, allowed to live only in public hotels, most contacts are carefully scrutinized, and those Chinese who dare to speak with them privately may be risking their political futures. Teachers of English, on the other hand, live within their workplace but are segregated with other foreign guests. From November 1979 to March 1980 we had the rare opportunity of living and working at a teaching hospital in central China that no foreigners had visited since before 1949. Although special accommodations were provided for our family, the nature of our work enabled us to become integrated, at least briefly, into the Chinese way of life.

Our chance to live and work in China came about as follows. In 1979, one of the authors, Myron S. Cohen, was a postdoctoral fellow in the Section of Infectious Disease at Yale University School of Medicine and the other, Gail E. Henderson, was a doctoral candidate in sociology at the University of Michigan with a strong background in Chinese studies and language. On 31 January 1979, during their visit to the United States, Vice-Premiers Deng Xiaoping and Fang Yi signed two major agreements on science and technology and cultural relations permitting the establishment of new exchange programs between the two nations. At Yale, interest in exchanges with China, and in medical exchanges in particular, was especially keen because of the university's long history of relations with the Medical

College in Changsha, Hunan Province. The Yale-China Association was eager to reestablish ties with this as well as other educational institutions in China. Furthermore, the cochairman of the Section of Infectious Disease, Dr. Richard K. Root, was favorably disposed to international exchanges and interested in pursuing a relationship with one or several medical colleges in China.

After the signing of the agreements, there remained a great deal of uncertainty about how to proceed in setting up an exchange. In the United States, the Committee on Scholarly Communications with the People's Republic of China (CSCPRC), under the National Academy of Sciences, was empowered to sponsor official projects and send a first group of American students to Beijing University. Yet it also seemed that the Chinese were open to other avenues of contact and that institution-to-institution exchanges would be acceptable. Initial communications with Chinese medical researchers were made by Dr. G. D. Hsiung, a well-known virologist at Yale and a trustee of the Yale-China Association, who had recently visited her birthplace, the city of Wuhan. With support from the Section of Infectious Disease, the Yale-China Association, and the University of Michigan Center for Chinese Studies, we agreed to conduct a feasibility study for future biomedical exchanges. After Dr. Hsiung had contacted several representatives there, it was agreed that the Hubei Provincial Medical College in Wuhan would be our host institution. Communications were difficult, and eight months elapsed before our visas were granted. In our letters, we requested housing near the medical college and provisions for the care of our infant daughter. Yet as we boarded the plane for Hong Kong and the train from Hong Kong to Wuhan, we had almost no idea what awaited us.

In fact what lay ahead were five uniquely difficult yet enriching months of experience. Although no foreigner can expect to understand Chinese society entirely, several factors combined to provide us with an especially good learning opportunity. First, we were in China at a time when the Communist regime was actively relaxing political control. Innovations in both politics and economics were blooming. In 1978, "Democracy Wall" in Beijing had proclaimed interest in a new kind of politics, and Deng's government seemed willing to endorse almost any kind of economic reform as long as it increased China's sagging productivity. Moreover, we went to a provincial capital a thousand miles south of Beijing, far from the seat of national power. The medical college and teaching hospital to which we were assigned had had no foreign visitors since before the Chinese revolution; as their test case, we were given much more freedom than those foreigners dealing with already established foreign affairs offices. Third, we had well-defined occupational roles in the unit; one of us functioned as a medical researcher, the other as an English teacher and translator. We lived in the hospital employees' housing complex, our daughter was cared for by a day-care teacher, and we established a routine largely similar to that of our neighbors and colleagues. Finally, we were a family in a very family-oriented society, and this fact probably contributed more than any other to our ability to relate to the people with whom we lived and worked.

In this book we attempt to achieve several goals. First, we describe what it is like to live and work in a Chinese *danwei*—a "work unit" or "workplace." In this case the *danwei* was a hospital, attached to a larger *danwei*, the medical college. Through descriptions of the function of this *danwei* and our own experiences in it, we aim to demonstrate the fundamental importance of this institution: the *danwei* touches every aspect of life in urban China. Second, we attempt to fit our observations into a sociological framework, with emphasis on key issues such as the options available to workers and professionals assigned to our institution. Finally, we describe the function of a medical school and hospital in the People's Republic of China. Worldwide attention has been focused on the health services system in China, and 10 percent of all organized tours to the country consist of physicians. Our observations are intended to broaden and strengthen American perceptions of medical care in China and to provide subsequent visitors with a helpful preview.

The book is organized to convey a sense of the work unit as a living organism and to stress the interrelationship between informal and formal life. Our coverage therefore moves from informal daily life inside the *danwei*, to the formal organization of work in the unit, to relations with the clients from outside the unit. This organization is also intended to emphasize the relative insularity of units such as the hospital. There is a real sense of being inside rather than outside the work unit, not only because there actually are walls around it but also because so much of life and work is dependent on the unit. To help create a solid impression of life and work in a *danwei*, one chapter in each of the three sections is devoted primarily to ethnographic description.

After a personal and historical overview in chapter 1, chapter 2 describes daily life in our *danwei*: the setting, daily routines, family life, housing, shopping, and holiday activities. Chapter 3 discusses the degree of control the work unit has over membership—that is, assignment to the unit and ability to exit from it—and the degree of separation of private from public life.

The second section is devoted to work in the *danwei*. Chapter 4 de scribes the routine of work on the infectious disease ward in the hospital, the setting, the various ward jobs, and the backgrounds of the people who work there. Chapter 5 places the ward and the hospital in the context of the larger administrative structure, with its hierarchy of management and finance; explores the role of leaders and the issue of work autonomy; and examines the impact of the unit on the power of professionals within the hospital, as well as the career mobility of unit staff.

The final section focuses on the clients of the *danwei*. Chapter 6 describes the system through which patients reach this particular referral hospital and presents a study of patients on the infectious disease ward. Chapter 7 examines the relationships between clients and practitioners, with emphasis again on how control is exercised and what strategies are developed to meet individual needs. Chapter 8 describes the delivery of medical care on the ward, with a focus on patients with whose care we became involved. Six appendixes present translations of charts that hung on the walls of the ward, outlining regulations for health care workers, and a list of lectures given to nurses. The last appendix discusses the methodology of our study.

Chapel Hill, North Carolina
February 1983

Acknowledgments

This book is the culmination of a journey to China with our infant daughter. We wish to thank Doctors G. D. Hsiung, Samuel O. Thier, Richard K. Root, John L. Morris, and John B. Starr, who helped make this opportunity possible. Marilyn and Richard Root volunteered their home to smooth our departure and return. The Department of Internal Medicine at Yale University, the Yale-China Association, the Hsiung Scholarship Fund, and the Center for Chinese Studies at the University of Michigan provided financial support for our journey. During part of the preparation of this book Gail Henderson was supported by an American Council of Learned Societies Mellon Fellowship.

Many friends and colleagues in the fields of sociology, sinology, and public health volunteered their time and insights. These include Doctors Robert H. Fletcher, Deborah Davis-Friedmann, Jean C. Oi, Andrew G. Walder, and Myron E. Wegman. Doctors William A. Fischer, Renée C. Fox, and G. D. Hsiung read the entire manuscript and provided invaluable comments. University of Michigan Professors Martin K. Whyte, Michel Oksenberg, Mayer N. Zald, and Robert E. Cole, as members of Gail Henderson's dissertation committee, helped shape the book from its inception. Michel Oksenberg actually visited our *danwei* in China, and his notion of the cellular nature of Chinese society helped us develop our own view of the role of the work unit. Perhaps most important was the contribution of Martin Whyte. Much of the sociological direction for this study originated with him, and through his own example of careful, thoughtful scholarship he helped us make the most of our experiences in China.

We wish to acknowledge the many people who helped prepare the manuscript, including Anne C. Weston, Annie Price, Dianne Buckner,

Frederick R. Henderson, and Audrey S. Henderson. Betty P. Lloyd created the illustrations. Ed Tripp at Yale University Press encouraged us from the beginning of this project; Ann Hawthorne skillfully edited the manuscript; and Charlotte Dihoff brought it to production.

Finally, we thank the members of the infectious disease ward and the hospital staff of the Second Attached Hospital of Hubei Provincial Medical College. These Chinese friends and colleagues are too numerous to list, but their kind reception of us and our daughter shaped our vision of their country. Furthermore, they provided us with the most indispensable requirement of Chinese life: a *danwei*, which we now think of as our own. We hope this work does justice to our *danwei*.

1

The *Danwei* and China: Setting the Stage

We arrived in Wuhan on 15 November 1979 and were greeted at the train station by a delegation of hospital and medical college officials, physicians, and nurses, most of whom would become important figures in our life in China. We were whisked away in a 1940s-style Shanghai-brand sedan to a military hotel on the shores of East Lake, where we stayed for three weeks while our hosts prepared our apartment. We learned that we had been assigned by the Chinese government to live and work at a teaching hospital attached to Hubei Provincial Medical College, both of which were located just down East Lake Road from our hotel. To our surprise and pleasure, we were given a staff apartment located on the hospital grounds. A cook was assigned from the patients' kitchen, and a day-care teacher from the hospital employees' nursery came to look after our daughter. We were provided with an office in the infectious disease ward, access to hospital and medical college officials, and tours of and more limited access to other hospitals in the area. All our needs were met within the walls of our work unit, or *danwei*, the Second Attached Hospital of Hubei Provincial Medical College.

In the thirty-five years since the founding of the People's Republic of China, the political environment has changed often. Most of these changes have stemmed from implementation of economic and social policies designed to emphasize egalitarianism during certain periods (the Great Leap Forward, 1958–1961; and the Cultural Revolution, 1966–1976) and economic development during others (the post-1949 Soviet influence, 1950–1958; the post–Great Leap Forward retrenchment, 1961–1966; and the post–Cultural Revolution era, 1976–present). These profound policy shifts reflect the dilemma faced by all modern socialist nations: how to maintain socialist ideals of equality while promoting modern, industrial development.

In China, the debate has manifested itself in experiments in a variety of modes of economic centralization and decentralization, in the redistribution of welfare and social service funds and personnel, and in the introduction of new policies in areas such as education and culture that were viewed as most closely tied with the creation of a correct socialist ideology. More radical periods have involved attempts to eliminate the advantages enjoyed by urban, technologically sophisticated "mental workers."

In 1976, Mao Zedong's death and the subsequent fall of the "Gang of Four" marked the end of a ten-year experiment in radical egalitarianism. During the Cultural Revolution, any institution, profession, ideology, or individual accused of fostering elitism was attacked. In education, recruiting practices were altered to favor children of workers, peasants, and soldiers, and curricula were curtailed and dramatically politicized. In industry, new participatory forms of management were introduced and material incentives

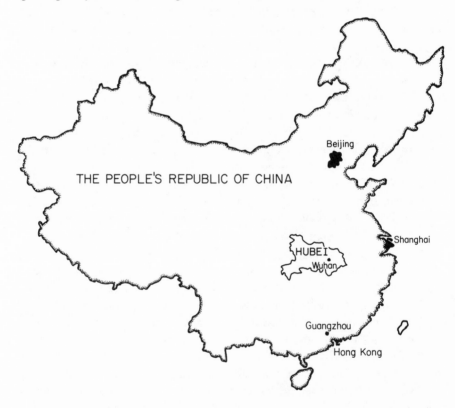

Figure 1. Wuhan, Hubei Province, People's Republic of China

decried as antisocialist. Intellectuals and administrators in most organizations, including the Chinese Communist party, were held accountable for the rise of a new privileged class and most were "sent down to the countryside" to be "reeducated" through physical labor and political discussion.

Events in medicine and public health were a microcosm of the larger political scenario. In the early years of the People's Republic of China, biomedical research received enormous attention. As a result of careful planning and political solution to public health issues, a variety of contagious diseases (such as venereal disease and trachoma) were eradicated. Certain areas of biomedical research received adequate funding to allow Chinese investigators to compete internationally. In this setting, Chinese scientists were the first to synthesize insulin, an accomplishment discussed in virtually every description of medicine in China (Horn 1969). Health care became a labor-intensive industry through the creation of a class of health care workers (later called "barefoot doctors") competent to deal with minor illnesses and, more important, to direct independent health campaigns at a local level. Likewise, traditional medical doctors, scorned by the Western-trained practitioners who were primarily responsible for health care policy and delivery before 1949 (Bowers 1972), were incorporated into this system.

Not surprisingly, during the Cultural Revolution medical practitioners and investigators were among those susceptible to the greatest criticism. The Ministry of Health was attacked for elitism, overreliance on Western techniques, and emphasis on urban development at the expense of the rural majority (Lampton 1977). Medical, nursing, and other training schools were shut down for several years, and many teachers and administrators were sent to the countryside to engage in more practical and politically relevant work. Basic science research ceased. Medical funds and personnel were redistributed and cooperative medical insurance programs introduced, to provide more equitable health care for the rural areas (Blendon 1979). Most urban hospitals rotated at least one-third of their staff to rural counties and communes. The barefoot doctors and other nonphysician health care workers became even more central to the system. Finally, in the urban hospitals, and in the medical schools as they gradually reopened, physicians, scientists, and administrators were criticized for elitism, and structural changes were introduced to undercut their dominance. Ranks were abolished. Overt signs of privilege (such as better housing and influence over placement of children in schools or jobs) were disallowed. There was sharing of tasks so that lower-level staff performed medical procedures and developed remarkable professional authority, whereas intellectuals were engaged in physical labor.

Above all, politics was emphasized to an extraordinary degree. When asked what it was like in the hospital during the Cultural Revolution, a physician responded, "We went to political meetings all the time."

Ironically, during this time of near chaos in the Chinese health care system, political relations between the United States and China improved sufficiently to allow Western investigators a firsthand look. The earliest surveyors may have been misled by the efforts of the Chinese to display only their best facilities and to avoid extensive contact with Western visitors (Leys 1977). Nevertheless, in the last ten years a considerable number of Western books and articles have been published describing, publicizing, advocating, and (rarely) criticizing the Chinese system of health care delivery (Blendon 1979; Bowers and Purcell 1974; Cheng 1973; Dimond 1971; Hsu 1971; Hu 1975; Lampton 1974, 1977, 1981; Mechanic and Kleinman 1980; New and New 1977; Quinn 1972; M. M. Rosenthal 1981; Sidel 1972; Sidel and Sidel 1973, 1982; U.S. Department of Health and Human Services 1980; Wegman, Lin, and Purcell 1973). Most of these assessments have been thoughtful and accurate, but they have been persistently limited by very brief and narrow access to the system.

By the time of our stay in China (November 1979–March 1980), most of the Cultural Revolution reforms had been dismantled. Vice-Premier Deng Xiaoping had reversed most of the radical policies in economics, culture, education, and health. The Gang of Four was blamed at every turn for China's stagnation. In stark contrast to the Cultural Revolution's subordination of production to politics, Deng's primary commitment was to raising productivity through the application of advanced technology, use of foreign input in economics and development, and employment of China's own technical experts in the nation's modernization drive. In a local setting such as the medical college and hospital units, these changes translated into fewer political meetings; greater emphasis on technical education of all types; the reintroduction of job ranks, promotions, and cash bonus incentives; and a positive attitude toward intellectuals, specialists, and the importance of their contributions. Some of these changes were still being implemented while we were there.

After moving into our apartment at the Second Attached Hospital, we established routines of work on the ward, teaching English, and attending various meetings and tours to learn more about our immediate environment. At every turn, we were increasingly impressed with how important the work unit was to other hospital staff and to us. For example, most patients reached the Second Attached Hospital only after referral from their own work units. The position of hospital staff, including professionals, was determined by the *danwei* system, which provided few job alternatives and placed the staff under the authority of work unit leaders. The *danwei* began to dominate our thoughts and conversations. As we talked with other foreigners in Wuhan, we heard about their work units and were able to make direct comparisons of physical structure, function, and, most important, the unit directors and administrators, to whom the Chinese and we referred as "our leaders."

The importance of the work unit lies primarily in its unique combination of social, political, and economic life—much like an "urban village." During the first decade of Communist rule, all workplaces in urban China (factories, schools, hospitals, stores, government offices) were organized into administrative units. This move was accompanied by the restriction of free migration into urban areas, the socialization of Chinese industry and commerce, and the centralization of job and housing assignment by the state. Each work unit was placed under the jurisdiction of its appropriate occupational bureaucracy—a hospital under the Ministry of Health, a university under the Ministry of Education. Units also are under the authority of other administrative bodies concerned with the allocation of personnel, the provision of services, and the maintenance of public security.

In addition to their economic role, work units became a convenient focus of political activities in Chinese cities. Since the establishment of the People's Republic, the Chinese Communists have relied heavily on a high level of political mobilization among their citizens to accomplish the transformation of the society into a socialist state (Hinton 1966, Barnett 1969). On the local level, mass campaigns to achieve economic, political, and social goals were conducted in the arena of the "small group" (*xiaozu*), a party-led organization composed of work unit members (or neighbors) and created for purposes of study, discussion, and other political activities (Whyte 1974). In the hospital, for example, there was at least one small group in each ward, and all met weekly to discuss national political issues and local concerns.

Work units are thus firmly embedded both in the economic hierarchy of a socialist government and in the parallel political administration of the Chinese Communist party. They are characterized by a fairly stable staff population, and the larger *danwei* also provide housing and other services. These factors combine to produce an intense and unique environment in which many functions of society and of family life take place. Figure 2 illustrates the relationship of the *danwei* to higher levels of authority and to work unit members.

Figure 3 locates the hospital work unit in its larger context. The hospital *danwei* is embedded in the Communist party, the Health Ministry bureaucracy, and the cultural framework of health care and health behavior in China. The hospital unit is responsible for the delivery of health care services to a patient population determined by the state. It is also responsible for housing and the provision of services for the majority of its staff, whose membership in the unit is also largely determined by the state. The hospital

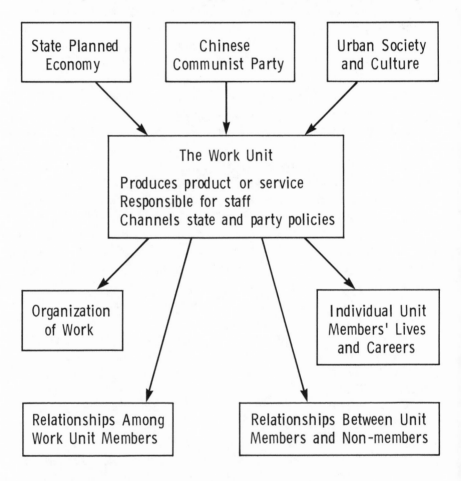

Figure 2. The Position of the Work Unit in Chinese Society

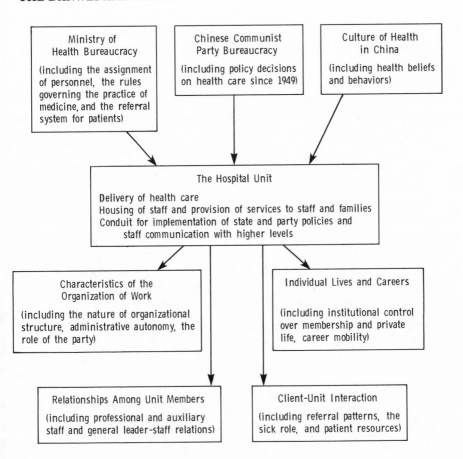

Figure 3. The Position of the Hospital Unit in Chinese Society

unit is the vehicle through which state and party health policies are implemented, and through which staff may communicate with higher-level authorities. Finally, this structural arrangement has a significant impact on the way in which the hospital actually functions, on relationships among staff, leaders, and patients, and on the lives and careers of the hospital personnel.

Danwei are isolated from each other in relatively closed systems, dependent upon higher levels for the source of their power and authority over members. The *danwei* system is, of course, not the sole force affecting the lives of work unit members. Other factors include the family, relationships with people outside the *danwei*, membership in neighborhood organizations, the power of the professional within a bureaucratic organization, con-

straints on middle-level leaders, and the influence of the Communist party
and other national organizations. Nevertheless, the *danwei* has an extraordinary influence on its individual members and (in our case) on the formal
and informal relations among the hospital administrators, doctors, nurses,
and patients. This influence does not lessen the importance of the other factors, but rather interacts with them and provides an additional layer of control with which Chinese citizens must cope in their daily lives.

Our work unit was a medium-sized *danwei*, a tertiary-care urban medical facility. Neither of these institutions has been adequately described in
the Western literature. Our experiences in the work unit repeatedly raised
several sociological questions that deserve focus and discussion.[1] The first
involves the nature of membership in the *danwei*. How are people assigned
to their unit? How do they leave? Second, how much organizational control
does the *danwei* exercise over its staff and clients? Is work tightly or loosely
organized? What aspects of unit members' private lives are subject to public
regulation? Finally, what are the dynamics of personal relationships within
work units and between staff and clients, and how are conflicts resolved?
These are not isolated topics. For example, when organizational membership is voluntary, people are generally less dependent on their organizations
and more confident in encounters with superiors than when fewer exit options are available.[2] On the other hand, leaders' authority over permanent

---

1. The questions are drawn from Erving Goffman's *Asylums* (1961), in which he describes
"total institutions," environments in which inmates sleep, play, and work together while being
denied contact with the outside world. We avoid explicit reference to the term *total institution*
for two reasons. First, although there are some similarities between Chinese work units and the
total institutions observed by Goffman, the latter are extreme examples of institutional control,
and as such, the term creates a frightening totalitarian image. Second, as Dr. Renée C. Fox
suggested in a thoughtful criticism of this manuscript, the total-institution model is limited by
cultural and social specificity. That is, Goffman's model is based on a Western conception of
the individual, the person, and the relationship between the individual and the group. In
China, on the other hand, the individual person is defined much more in terms of a social context, a matrix of human relationships. Consequently, although we address sociological questions about the relationship between the individual and the institution, we eschew a label that
may blind us to the reality of the experience from the Chinese point of view.

2. This truism of organizational behavior is brilliantly elucidated in Albert O. Hirschman's *Exit, Voice, and Loyalty* (1970). Hirschman proposed that when people are dissatisfied
with an organization or product they either exit or voice their grievances, and that these
choices are influenced by a third factor, loyalty. Hirschman's paradigm is based on a market
economy in which exit is a realistic option. In Chinese work units, however, membership is
rarely voluntary, and thus exit is seldom an option. Hirschman postulated that in such cases,
voice would be used more frequently. Others who have studied consumer response in nonmarket economies (Kolarska and Aldrich 1980) have questioned this assertion, and certainly Goffman's descriptions of inmates in total institutions do not portray heightened use of voice to

employees may be surprisingly limited if the environment is organized to provide effective feedback strategies. On paper, the regulations of the *danwei* create a rigid and comprehensive system of life and work. In practice, though still awesome in scope, this new form of Communist organization has blended closely with older, traditional styles of organizational behavior in China.

---

express dissatisfaction as a result of their lack of an exit option. Despite these criticisms, Hirschman's initial juxtaposition of exit and voice alerts us to the possible relationship between these two responses to an organization (see chapter 5).

For a discussion of organizational dependency brought about by lack of alternative sources for satisfaction of needs, see Stinchcombe (1970).

2

Daily Life in the *Danwei*

The hospital complex (see figure 4), its staff dormitories, and various auxiliary buildings are located by a lake on the outskirts of the fifth largest city in China, Wuhan.[1] As a teaching hospital, it serves the needs of the medical college, which is adjacent to the hospital grounds. As a provincial-level hospital, it treats patients referred from fifteen counties in the province, with a combined population of some 7 million. The total population of the province is 33 million.

There are several entrances to the hospital *danwei* from the main road, which winds along the lake. Unmarked gateways and some well-trodden dirt paths lead to apartment buildings of varying style, height, and age. Farther down the road, the main entrance gate exhibits a black and white sign, "SECOND ATTACHED HOSPITAL OF HUBEI PROVINCIAL MEDICAL COLLEGE UNDER THE ADMINISTRATION OF THE PROVINCIAL BUREAU OF HEALTH." Heavy wrought-iron gates hang on either side of an eight-foot wall that gives the impression of encircling the entire hospital complex.

From the front gate, a short road ends in a circular driveway in front of the main hospital building. A tall pine tree in the center of the driveway obscures the view of a four-story, Soviet-style hospital constructed of graying cement during the fifties. Jeeps, Shanghai-brand sedans, white ambulances, bikes, hand-pulled carts containing produce or patients, and a variety of people dressed in either white coats or the ubiquitous dark-blue, gray, or army green populate the drive at all times. The pace is unhurried. In warm weather, benches are brought outside for hospital staff to sun themselves on

---

1. Wuhan comprises the three cities of Wuchang, Hankou, and Hanyang, located at the junction of the Han and Yangzi rivers.

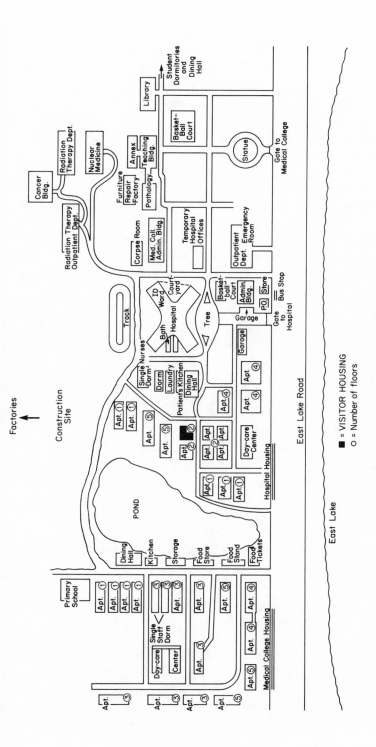

Figure 4. Hubei Provincial Medical College and the Second Attached Hospital

the steps. Peasants arrive to sell their vegetables or fruit, and news of unusual items for sale quickly spreads through the hospital. Except on the coldest days, an old vendor stands beside the front door offering visitors a final chance to purchase bread, cookies, and cigarettes.

Outside the front gate, more people wait at the bus stop to be taken to the city or to the nearby countryside. The buses are white and blue, and often two are joined by an accordionlike black material that looks as if it should expand and contract as the crowds push in and out in massive numbers. Behind the bus stop are a green post office, housing its worker and his family in the back, and a small food store. In front of this store, a tiny old woman with few remaining teeth sets up a fire pot and wok to sell a kind of deep-fried bread (*mianwo*) that is a local speciality. When it rains, she cooks with one hand and holds her umbrella with the other.

The hospital is surrounded by low bushes that often function as natural clotheslines for patients or their relatives to dry freshly washed clothes. Occasionally the garments are little more than tatters, but they are repeatedly washed and dried until the last bit of usefulness is pounded out of them. The hospital grounds consist of packed dirt and low-lying shrubs or small pine trees. Near the medical college are several wooded sections in which medical students pace back and forth with books in hand. At the slightest rain, the grounds become impassable. Cement sidewalks and narrow roads wind around the hospital and back by all the staff apartments so that a jeep or truck can reach most sections.

As one faces the hospital, the staff apartments are to the left, specialized or newly constructed facilities at the back, and the medical college on the right. Bricks lie in large and small piles in every empty lot, tangible evidence of the constantly changing physical environment. In the midst of the bricks, chickens scratch, children create makeshift platforms for table tennis, and construction teams are rarely absent. The apartment buildings are brick and cement. The older ones are one story high, with communal kitchens and baths for several families in individual three-room apartments. The newest buildings are four- and five-story cement structures housing one hundred families. In addition to housing, the unit includes a dining hall, a day-care center, a bathhouse attached to the hospital boiler room, an administrative office, a garage for unit cars and jeeps, and shops for the maintenance and repair staff (plumbers, carpenters, electricians). Behind the hospital, construction of a new pharmaceutical factory is under way. From this point it takes no more than five or ten minutes to walk to the front of the unit.

The medical college facilities are spread over a campus slightly larger than the hospital grounds. They include several teaching buildings, a library, student dormitories, a dining hall, an athletic field, administrative offices, and several small college-run industries. Because land is scarce even on the outskirts of the city, the housing, dining hall, food store, day-care center, and primary school for the medical college staff are all located on the other side of the hospital grounds, beyond the hospital staff apartments.

Not all of the approximately 830 people who work at the hospital live in the *danwei*. Some live with parents or spouses in other work units and travel each day by bus or bicycle, sometimes commuting as much as an hour each way. Likewise, not all the people in each household work in the *danwei*. Some spouses or children leave the unit each morning for employment elsewhere. However, approximately two-thirds of those who work in the hospital live in the hospital's apartments or single staff dormitories, and many spouses and even some children are employed by the *danwei*. The walls and gates and the close proximity of most services create an atmosphere of people working and living together in a somewhat closed community. The profusion of shared experiences, the necessary cooperation, and the routines performed by all sharpen the sense of community.

The daily rhythm of routine events creates a backdrop for the larger dramas of life and work. Very early each morning, the individually and collectively raised chickens combine their voices in a discordant chorus calling all to rise. For breakfast, most people send one member of the family out to the dining hall to pick up steamed bread, oil cakes, or dumplings. Those too late for a family meal will munch their breakfast on the short walk to the hospital. People carrying kettles and thermoses line up at the hospital boiled-water faucet, which is directly attached to the boiler room. A sign over the faucet praises the hospital for providing such a convenience to its staff. Occasionally a woman waits with a metal pan and tiny stool or chair, preparing to wash out some clothes or perhaps quickly wash her own hair in the hot-water drain, which runs alongside the drinking-water faucet. After breakfast, mothers and fathers carry their tightly bundled children to the day-care center. Even in mild weather, the children are wrapped in several layers of blankets, quilts, and padded clothing. Toddlers are led by the hand, and school-age children dressed in colorful jackets walk with playmates and neighbors to the primary school, which serves the families of both the hospital and the medical school staff. The local high school is a ten-minute walk down the main road that runs along the lake.

By eight, everyone has disappeared except the logistics or service staff (*houqing*), who are getting food and laundry ready for the day, and a few grandparents tending young children in an apartment courtyard. Periodically, the morning silence is broken by the sounds of construction teams moving bricks from their stacks in empty lots to some new project in the unit. These unskilled workers are often young men and women waiting for job assignments by the state. Their main task is to pile bricks into wheelbarrows and push, pull, or run downhill with them in an effort to keep them under control and moving toward the construction site. As they pick up speed, the wheelbarrows sometimes get away from the young workers, overturning in a crash of bricks at the bottom of the hill. Everyone knows to keep out of the path of the speeding wheelbarrows.

At noon, people pour out of the buildings and stop by the dining hall to purchase a square-shaped portion of rice or several squares for a family. The portions never seem to fit well into the rectangular metal containers used as food plates, and the large rice squares protrude precariously as people rush out. To avoid the ten- or fifteen-minute wait for lunch, some carry their rice home and cook vegetables in their own kitchens. Others, for convenience and to save home fuel, buy their lunch and either take it home or eat it at the dining hall. Food coupons are sold by the dining hall accountant each month for use only at a prescribed eating place, and only this currency can be used. In addition, government ration coupons for items such as wheat and sugar are required at dining halls and stores. An individual may eat modestly at the dining hall for 20 yuan a month (U.S. $13.20) or very well for 30–40 yuan.[2] Most agree that home cooking is better and a little cheaper, but the dining hall is chosen for convenience.

Directly after the noon meal, everyone not on duty lies down for an hour's rest (*xiuxi*). In the heat of summer, this nap may extend to two hours. Primary school children are home, but the day-care youngsters take their naps at the center from noon until three. The *danwei* is very quiet until about half past one, when people begin to stir and get ready to go back to work or school by two. People who live in other nearby work units usually ride their bicycles home for lunch and a rest. Those who live too far away may lie down in the on-call room or visit with friends. Some take noon duty more frequently so that they can leave earlier in the afternoon.

Except for those people on evening or night shifts, the work day ends around five or half past five. At that time, the hospital staff stroll back to their homes. Parents pick up their babies and young children from the day-care center, where the older ones are dressed in their coats and hats, sitting

2. An exchange rate of $1.00 U.S. = 1.50 yuan is used.

in neat semicircles. A long line forms at the hot-water faucet. Families with a newspaper on order send one member to the front gate office, where unit mail, journals, and newspapers are received. If the weather permits, children play on the sidewalks until they are called for dinner. Evening meals are often prepared at home, especially in families in which a mother or mother-in-law is home to begin preparations early. Those with busy schedules or night duty take advantage of dining hall services, and staff working all night are given another meal at ten. Children whose parents are away for the night often stay at home alone. There are some "latchkey" children in the unit, but neighbors are at most only a shout away, and from the age of eight or ten, children are left alone.

After supper things quiet down. In pleasant weather, families may go for a walk or sit out on their balconies. Children are put to bed, and many adults engage in some sort of studying. When there is an outdoor movie, families can be seen at twilight, each member carrying a stool or chair to sit on during the show. Families with television sets are visited by those without. In general, evenings are uneventful, and people are in bed between ten and eleven. The only sound ever to disturb our night's sleep (besides our own daughter's cries) was the screeching of a wild cat in heat.

This *danwei* is located in a city but retains some of the same dependence upon the vagaries of climate and temperature as its rural counterparts. An arbitrary judgment made in an earlier era and upheld by the current regime decreed that any part of China north of the Yangzi River is northern in climate, and everything south of the Yangzi is warm. Thus home heating is subsidized only in the "northern" regions. Our hospital is located in the part of Wuhan that lies south of the Yangzi, and during the light winter snowfalls it is difficult to subscribe to the notion that one lives in a southern climate. During the winter many of the *danwei* staff have little or no indoor heat; indoor and outdoor clothing become indistinguishable. In the evenings, to cook and to warm themselves, people use coal stoves, and the level of carbon monoxide in the air rises alarmingly. Day-care centers, schools, and businesses located in small, closed-in areas pipe the fumes out a window or roof. The hospital does maintain a low level of steam heat in the wards, for which patients are charged .02 yuan per day, but higher temperatures are reserved for operating rooms and newborn care.

Sunny days are thus a commodity. Laundry is usually done on the one day off each week. In our *danwei*, this is Sunday, but the days are staggered throughout the city to ease the inevitable congestion in stores and markets. But no matter what day of the week, when the sun comes out, clothes, quilts, and pillows appear on the balconies of many apartments. Those few without balconies hang the wash on bamboo poles eased carefully out windows and doors. People bring small chairs outside to sit by a southern wall and warm themselves. Any housework that can be done outdoors is brought along.

Wuhan's climate in the summer has earned it the name "the oven of China." Padded clothing is shed for light, loose-fitting cotton shirts, skirts, and trousers. Movement slows. People stay indoors, out of the sun, and depend on fans and the cooling touch of bamboo beds, which are used during the three hottest months. At night, gauze netting protects against mosquitoes. Young people swim and boat in the lake across from the hospital, and ice cones are sold at the bus stop. Between the cold of the winter and heat of the summer there may be a few weeks of spring and a few more of autumn. But the weather of Wuhan is lamented by all, especially by those who have been relocated from more favorable climates.

Rain or shine, summer or winter, family shopping needs persist. Primary among the duties of all family members is the periodic (often daily) marketing trip. For the purchase of large consumer items and specialty goods, staff from our *danwei* board the bus for Wuchang or Hankou early Sunday morning. This trip, however, takes an entire day, so errands are generally saved for monthly expeditions. Most of the daily necessities, such as food, toilet articles, dry goods, and clothing, are available at the neighborhood market, the Fruit Lake Stores.

It takes five minutes to bicycle to Fruit Lake, ten to fifteen to walk. Most people ride their bikes and then walk back, pushing vehicles heavily laden with produce. The asphalt road winds along the shore of the lake, with new construction sites rapidly popping up between brilliant green rice fields. The road is divided by a white line made of tiny bits of broken porcelain, laid neatly together in an endless mosaic. On the way to the stores, one passes the dormitories of the medical college and those of another work unit, a large factory that makes machine tools. When we make this journey no one recognizes us, and many more people stare. The shopping district includes a produce store, a butcher shop, a camera store, a tailor, a dumpling (*baozi*) stand, a yarn-producing textile factory, a very small branch of New China Bookstore (Xinhua Shudian), a post office, a department store (which was closed when a new four-story department store opened at the end of the street), and a multitude of peddlers, vendors, and repair people lining the sidewalks.

Even on weekdays, Fruit Lake bustles with activity. On Sundays it is difficult to pass through the crowds. At the top of the street, buses stop and trolley cars turn around to make their way back to the city. At the other end of the street, a large red gate and imposing sign mark the grounds of the Hubei provincial government offices. Perhaps because of the proximity to the provincial capital, People's Liberation Army uniforms fill the street. Dark blue and green are broken by an occasional cheerful jacket. Girls wear printed shirts and scarves. The road and sidewalk are dusty or muddy, depending on the weather. When the trucks come in from the neighboring communes, mounds of produce—especially cabbage—are dumped upon the sidewalk, forcing people to make detours into the street. People of all ages mingle, play, push, and stroll.

Perhaps the most distinctive aspect of shopping in China is the sense of chance involved in any expedition. One never knows what will be available. Was there good cabbage last week? That does not mean there will be any this week. Did Comrade Li see a warm winter hat in the department store a few days ago? It may or may not still be on the shelves. Salespeople cannot predict what will be coming in or when. Connections are bad on the telephone and only a few people have one, so it is not common to phone ahead for information. Thus consumers set out shopping ready for anything, particularly sales. News of a special sale or the availability of hard-to-get items spreads quickly. Lines form, and people buy items like shoes, handbags, or a special kind of food for friends and relatives as well as for themselves. The limited availability of goods often seems to be a greater deterrent to purchase than whether or not one has enough money to buy them. People we knew saved money and spent it very carefully after thoughtful, comparative shopping. Yet often it seemed that they could not get what they wanted or had to wait for years to be given a coupon to purchase something in great demand (such as a Shanghai television or a bicycle).

Sundays are also a time to visit family and friends who live at a distance from the *danwei*. It is a great day for outings in the park, picture taking, and a family meal with grandparents. Those without extended family in or near the city are lonely on Sunday.

Other forms of entertainment include movies (the most popular diversion in China today) and the periodic acrobatic and performing acts that travel from town to town. At one variety show held at New Year's, the audience was treated to a potpourri of ideological messages—national minority dancing, Puccini arias sung by a Chinese woman dressed in a flowing blue chiffon gown, "Jingle Bells," and Chinese political tunes such as "Without the Chinese Communist Party, There Would Be No New China."

Televisions are now appearing both in the homes of unit staff and in the hospital wards. There are several stations, which broadcast from seven to ten each night, with educational shows in the morning. The evening programs usually include opera, variety shows, and movies—often those currently being shown in the movie houses.

SPRING FESTIVAL

Of all the Chinese holidays, Spring Festival—otherwise known as Chinese New Year's—is the most important. It is Thanksgiving, Christmas, New Year's, and Easter all rolled into one grand celebration. We were told that Spring Festival the year we were in China was the best it had been since before the Cultural Revolution. Produce and special New Year's foods poured in from the countryside. Oranges were available again; apparently it had been a capitalist crime to grow them during the Cultural Revolution. *Sutang*, a flaky candy that seems to be 99.9 percent sugar, had been rare in previous years, but this year (although it was still rationed) there was more than enough for everyone. Workers around the city were receiving New Year's bonuses, some as much as one or two months' salary (100 yuan). The hospital gave its workers 15–25 yuan apiece, depending on the amount of sick leave and vacation time taken, as well as special gifts to workers with very low salaries. The medical college gave 25 yuan to all staff.

The most common form of entertainment at Spring Festival is visiting friends and relatives. It takes weeks to prepare for the event. Even a month beforehand, the streets of Wuhan are more crowded than usual—so crowded that our *danwei* leaders advised us not to travel downtown. Everywhere we went we saw food being prepared, quilts aired, and vendors hawking a wide variety of goods. Even the hospital wards get a good spring cleaning by all the staff. It seems that the women work harder than the men at this time of year, and the women we asked about this agreed that the holidays were an extra burden for them.

The night before New Year's, everyone stays up late. In days past, people stayed up to watch for the "Nien Monster," to make sure he didn't eat some unsuspecting child; and then on New Year's, they went out to congratulate each other on not being eaten. Now, people watch fireworks and television. Fireworks were banned during the Cultural Revolution because they were considered a "waste of money," but they have returned in full force.

On New Year's day, everyone puts on new clothes and goes calling or receives callers. It is an exhausting round of parties and moviegoing, and of seeing friends and relatives one has not seen for a long time. The Central Broadcasting Station fills the entire day with a show featuring the top fifteen tunes of the year, which are carefully recorded on home tape recorders. The *danwei* workers' union buys movie tickets for staff, and theaters schedule the best entertainment.[3] The unit dining hall prepares a free meal for all who must eat alone on New Year's. People are given four days' vacation (two weeks if they must travel a long way to visit their families), and they fill the streets in a constant stream of activity and anticipation. Partly because of the long holiday, many young people get married at Spring Festival. In rural China, weddings still constitute a considerable financial burden (Parish and Whyte 1978), but in the cities these ceremonies seem to be less extravagant. The couple may have dinner with family and friends. Then, following a brief honeymoon trip, they are "at home" for several weeks in their new living quarters. Friends feel free to drop by unannounced and look at the wedding gifts, a practice not entirely appealing to the newlyweds.

In addition to the holiday celebrations at home, the unit itself and the work groups of the *danwei* hold Spring Festival parties. These are highly entertaining, often ritualized affairs.

The English department party began at nine in the morning, several days before Spring Festival. All the desks in the teachers' office were pushed together and covered with blue-and-white tablecloths, teacups, sesame snacks, cookies, candy peanuts, and watermelon seeds. We all sat around the table, and the head of the department gave a speech (mostly about us) and then we foreigners gave a speech (mostly about them) and presented them with some pictures for the office walls. Then one of the teachers, acting as master of ceremonies, explained the meaning of Spring Festival and announced that there would be "free talk." During this time, each person was required to give a short speech and a performance. Most of the performances ran to singing "do-re-mi" or Chinese opera. We sang "America the Beautiful" and a popular Chinese tune, "Tomorrow Will Be Sweet," complete with tambourine and kazoo. One teacher sang a World War II song: "We had no food or clothes, but the enemy gave us some; we had no guns or cannons, but the enemy gave us some." Finally, we played games, mostly number games or simple rhythm games in which each person coughs or

3. The workers' union is a mass organization open to all but capitalists. If one joins, and most do, .5 percent of one's monthly salary is deducted and matched by contributions from the government, for the unit welfare fund. This sum is used for sports, recreation, and other welfare activities.

claps a certain number of times in turn, and the one who makes a mistake must give a performance. The chance to see one's colleagues make fools of themselves in these performances was captivating. Two middle-aged women who were good friends and always sat near each other found the skits and off-tune singing so comical that they literally fell out of their chairs with mirth. We could not help but be caught up in the spirit of sharing good times with friends.

A much more boisterous affair was held two nights before New Year's at the unit dining hall—transformed by the workers' union into a carnival of balloons, streamers, games, good things to eat, and table-tennis competitions. Everyone in the *danwei* and all their children came. There was barely room to breathe. Booths featured pin the tail on the pig, ring toss, fish for fish, and other familiar events. Small prizes were offered. Children were wild to try everything. It was the night for the local table-tennis and pool champions to shine as they defended their titles against all challengers. The noise lasted late into the night.

HOUSING AND FAMILY LIFE

Even when one is assigned to work in an urban *danwei*, housing at that work unit is not guaranteed. Many *danwei*, particularly in crowded cities such as Shanghai or Guangzhou (Canton), have simply run out of room for staff dormitories. In these cases, people live in urban neighborhoods and commute to work. Housing in our *danwei* is said to be typical of factories, schools, and city and county hospitals in less congested urban areas. Approximately two-thirds of the hospital staff live on the grounds, and it is estimated that 70 to 80 percent of all hospital and medical staff are married to each other.

It is certainly more efficient for the work unit to house couples who work for the hospital or its parent and neighbor organization, the medical college.[4] Physicians and researchers who meet in school can logically be assigned to the same type of work unit. Likewise, among staff such as low-level administrators, service personnel, or workers in the unit's auxiliary organizations, a strong attempt is made to find work for both spouses or to give them both training for jobs in the same *danwei*. It is not uncommon for single people assigned to the unit to pair off and marry. There seemed

---

4. There have been recent conferences trying to arrange transfers to reunite separated spouses. See Foreign Broadcast Information Service, *Daily Report of the People's Republic of China*, 3 November 1980, 1–23.

to be a feeling that, as one person put it, it was "not appropriate for people of unequal education to marry." This sentiment was borne out in our observations of young people with similar occupations and educational degrees pairing up, as well as the very common occurrence of husbands and wives having the same or similar occupations.

In many countries, the size and location of one's housing is testimony to one's status. In China such distinctions may be true to some extent, but they are complicated by several factors. First, the only immediately apparent segregation in our *danwei* was that between single and married people. In a family-oriented society such as China, unmarried people may be its most disadvantaged minority. Their dormitories are sex segregated, with up to three persons living in a rather small room at a cost of about one yuan per person per month. A new staff member who is bringing a family, even if the spouse also works at the unit, must wait years to be assigned housing, in some cases as much as ten years. In the meantime, the couple may live in the spouse's unit, find a room with parents, or occasionally live separately until housing is found. In our *danwei*, the major determinants in obtaining an assignment to "nice" housing seemed to be length of association with the unit, luck, a policy to restore those persecuted during the Cultural Revolution to the equivalent of their previous quarters, and probably connections with the *danwei* leadership or housing office. Thus it was not at all uncommon to find doctors living next door to cooks or hospital maintenance workers. The director of the hospital, for example, lived in an apartment below a garage mechanic. Perhaps in response to earlier abuses by officials, the *danwei* administrators maintained a low profile in terms of housing. While we were there, they even moved out of their offices and worked in temporary structures in order to provide more space for unit members who had been waiting years to be assigned housing.

We were often told that living conditions in our *danwei* were better than those of other urban settings. Most of the apartment buildings have been constructed since 1949, and two new apartment buildings had just been completed. The standard apartment, for which families pay about five yuan per month, consists of an eating area, two bedrooms, and a small kitchen and bathroom (see figure 5).[5] The parents' bedroom usually doubles as a living room. An attempt is made to place larger families in more substantial apartments, but because most apartments have the same number of rooms, people with many children simply devise means to accommodate them within limited space. When children are young, they sleep with their

5. Of the five yuan, two are for rent and three are for utilities.

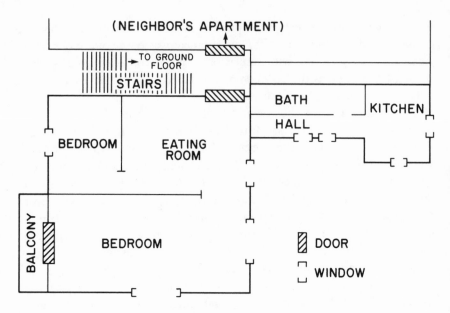

Figure 5. Floor Plan of a Typical Apartment in the Hospital Unit

parents. As they grow older, children may share beds; one family we knew with three boys in one room constructed bunk beds. When the eldest children are old enough for job assignment, they may obtain housing in other *danwei* or live with relatives. As children begin to find their own mates, the second bedroom often becomes the room for a married son and perhaps a grandchild.

For children of the *danwei* staff, this process of selecting a marriage partner, being assigned a job, and obtaining housing defies simple generalizations. Each family—and it is still the family rather than the individual that is considered of primary importance—works with a complex constellation of factors. These factors, discussed in detail in the next chapter, have changed considerably over time. Nevertheless, our observations produced some tentative conclusions.

The young people in our *danwei* generally seemed to live with their parents at least until they married, and often after marriage as well. One unmarried friend still living at home said, "Kids are kids for longer. I'm twenty-four and my parents still want to know where I am at night." In addition to parental attitudes and needs and the logistics of housing, there are other factors that influence marriage plans and prevent young people from

moving away from their parents at an early age. First, the state strongly rec-
ommends late marriage as part of the family planning program. Second, it
takes a long time to save enough money to set up an independent household. Couples may meet in their early twenties and save for several years before being able to purchase towels, sheets, furniture, and other expensive
consumer items. Couples commonly meet at school, in the neighborhood,
or at work. School officials frown upon student romances, in part because
of the late marriage rule and in part because they create difficulties for subsequent assignments to work units. For men and women in their mid-
twenties who do not seem to be meeting a mate on schedule, friends often
perform the traditional matchmaker role.[6] From such introductions and a
few dates, they must form opinions that may bind them to matrimony.
There is not a great deal of dating several people. A relationship that persists for a year or two invariably leads to marriage.

Once children are married, it is common to encounter three generations under one roof. A young teacher described the arrangements as "se-
quential" extended families. That is, the first child marries and moves in
with his parents while the second lives in a dormitory or at home. When the
second child marries, the first may move out. The youngest may end up living with the parents the longest. This arrangement seems to occur less commonly with married daughters than with sons; most women either move in
with their husband's family or set up individual households. Whether the
children are able to live with their parents or not, both the state and prevailing cultural norms dictate that children take an active responsibility for their
parents in old age.

Although these living arrangements in the *danwei* resemble the traditional Chinese family pattern, there have been important changes. First,
sheer physical constraints of urban living dictate smaller families. Second,
there has been a fundamental shift in power within the family from the
older to the younger generation. Part of this change is the result of the new
role of women as productive members of society. Because most women are
employed outside the home, household chores and child care are shared to
some extent by husbands or are performed by grandparents, particularly
grandmothers. Day care is available and is used by those without grandparents in the home; many feel, however, that a young infant is better off under the care of grandparents. In fact, in our unit several parents with very

6. Public matchmaking services have also recently been established in eighteen of the
twenty provinces, municipalities, and autonomous regions of China, including Beijing, Shanghai, and Tianjin. See "A Matchmaking Service," *Women of China*, April 1981, 39–40.

demanding schedules had sent their children to live with grandparents in the countryside or in distant cities rather than try to keep them at home. For a working woman, having a grandparent at home is definitely a help,[7] and the allotment of household tasks reflects, in part, the value of the young woman's earning power.

On the other hand, many elderly Chinese still maintain their respected position in the family. One middle-aged scientist described his relationship with his seventy-year-old father in unequivocal terms: "My father is still the master of our house and I am a child before him." In fact, power within the family may not shift to the younger generation if the grandparent continues to work into his or her retirement years. Such prolonged service occurs commonly among intellectuals and administrators, such as physicians and medical educators, on whose productive labor the administration continues to depend. Furthermore, many urban elderly now benefit from the state pension plan and even after retirement have their own sometimes considerable sources of income.[8] Thus, although many parents wish to live with their children, it may not be necessary for them to do so, and to take over perhaps undesirable household responsibilities.

The following sketches describe two families and their housing in our unit.

XIAO GONGREN: LITTLE WORKER

Xiao Gongren is a twenty-four-year-old cook.[9] He has grown up living in an apartment on the hospital grounds. His father, age sixty-six, works for the hospital *danwei* as a mechanic, maintaining the unit's jeeps and cars. His mother is a retired seamstress who also worked for the hospital making uniforms and other linens. He is the youngest of five children. His sister, a nurse, and her surgeon husband also live and work in the hospital unit. His mother cares for his sister's three-year-old daughter during the day, and often at night as well, for the parents are frequently on night duty at the hospital. His oldest brother is married and lives in another part of the city. Xiao Gongren and his two unmarried brothers share one bedroom, sleeping on

7. The presence of a grandparent may not, however, be a boon to the private, emotional life of the family. During our stay, conflict in our unit between a mother-in-law and daughter-in-law resulted in the suicide of the latter.

8. Deborah Davis-Friedmann (1981) has pointed out that those elderly with state pensions may constitute a privileged minority status group.

9. *Xiao* ("little") is a common term of address connoting familiarity as well as low status.

twin beds and a bunk bed that he laughingly labels the "fifth floor" of their four-story apartment building. One of the brothers works in the hospital *danwei* as a driver, and the other is a worker in a nearby college. Xiao Gongren's parents' bedroom doubles as a living room during the day. The apartment also has a kitchen, eating room, and bathroom.

Xiao Gongren was ten when the Cultural Revolution began, and he says that during this decade he sometimes went to school and sometimes did not. Even when he did, there was not much learning going on. As a result, his formal education went barely beyond grade school. He feels perplexed by the loss of his education, saying he does not understand why it all happened. He was assigned to work in the kitchen, which prepares food for hospital patients, about five years ago. Along with eight other apprentices, four men and four women, he is learning the art from a master chef, for whom he feels great respect and affection. Xiao Gongren is paid forty yuan each month, a portion of which he gives to his family. His rent is negligible and he gets all his meals free in the kitchen, so he feels quite well off. His social life revolves around friends and family in the *danwei*, as well as friends from school days and others who lived at the unit but have moved away. When he is twenty-five he plans to marry a girl who also lives and works in the *danwei*.

WAIKE YISHENG: SURGEON

Waike Yisheng is the chief of surgery at our hospital. His wife is also called "doctor," but more as an honorific title, for she received only two years' training at a technical high school. She works in the clinic of the large machine-tools factory near our work unit, riding her bicycle there each day. They are both from Wuhan, and they have three children. The oldest son is married and lives and teaches at the Chinese Technical Institute, about an hour's bus ride from the hospital. The daughter is twenty-eight and expecting her first child. She works as a radiological technician at a hospital in the city, and she and her new husband have moved into housing at that unit. As part of the national family planning program, they have pledged to have only one child and will receive housing, medical, educational, and food- and cloth-rationing benefits from their *danwei*. The youngest son is a worker at the same factory that employs his mother. During the day, he studies mechanical engineering as a part of a small group of workers in his factory who passed an examination to continue their education. Until his sister married, he lived in a dormitory at the factory because there was not enough room for both to sleep in his parents' apartment. Now he will probably move back.

The surgeon and his wife have a combined monthly income of over 150 yuan. Their apartment consists of two bedrooms, a kitchen, a bathroom, and a rather spacious eating room, for which they pay about five yuan a month. A white chicken resides under their kitchen sink and, much like a family pet, is let out each morning, walks down the flight of stairs to scratch in the dirt outside the apartment building, and in the evening marches home back up the stairs. Their living standard seems quite comfortable, perhaps because their children are grown and self-supporting. They have a television and plan to purchase a washing machine.

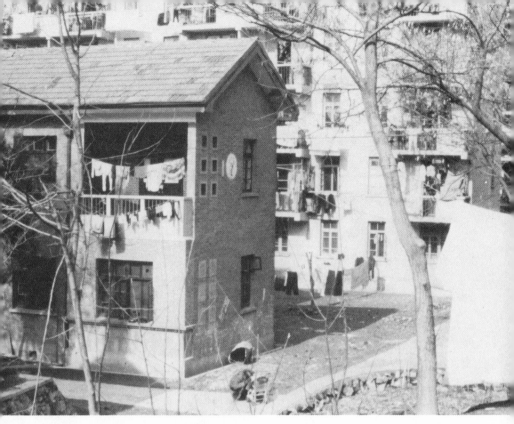

Our apartment (foreground, upper right).

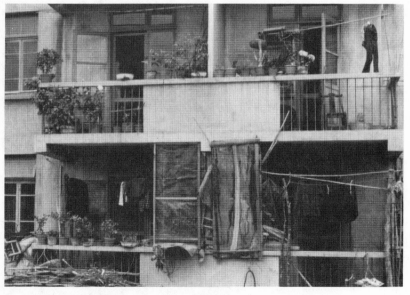

View from our apartment window emphasizes the use of balconies.

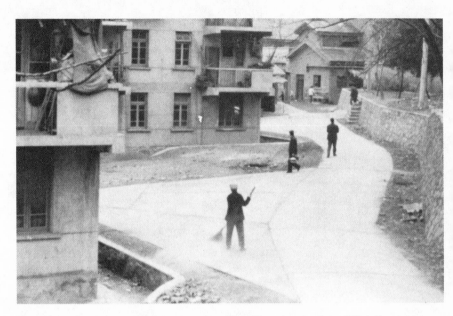

An older woman in our unit sweeps the sidewalk each morning. Officially retired unit members participate in a variety of volunteer activities.

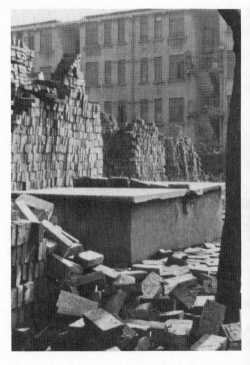

A ping pong table created for use by neighborhood children from available materials at a construction site near our apartment. An official wooden table was also available for tournaments.

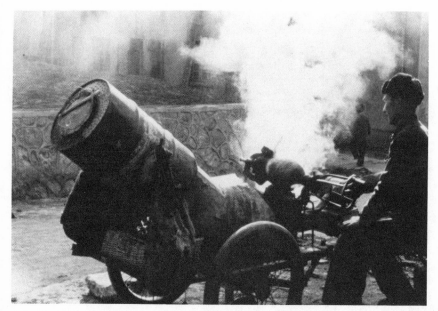

A local entrepreneur, who visited our unit once each week, "puffs" rice. He carried a license issued by the provincial government.

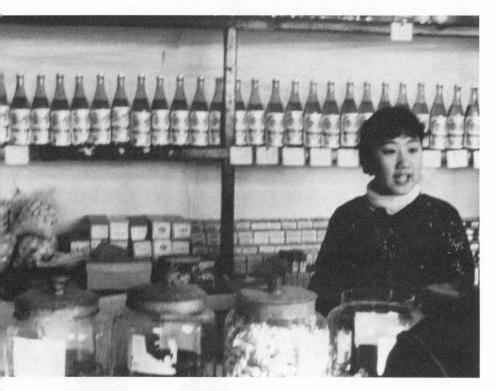

A *danwei* store, which stocks a basic but reliable supply of goods including condiments, toothpaste, toilet paper, and fruit in season.

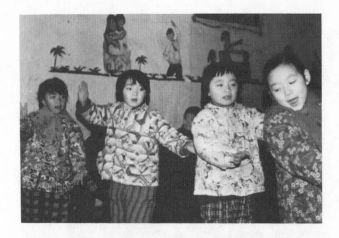

Children at the
hospital day care
center entertain
visitors.

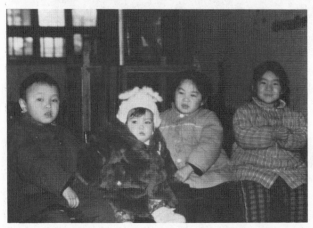

Our daughter, Jessie,
visits the day
care center.

A child at the day care center.

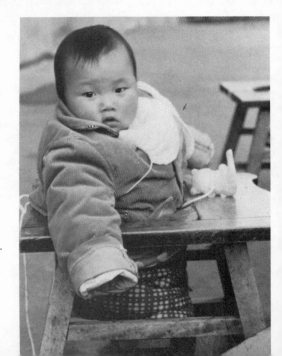

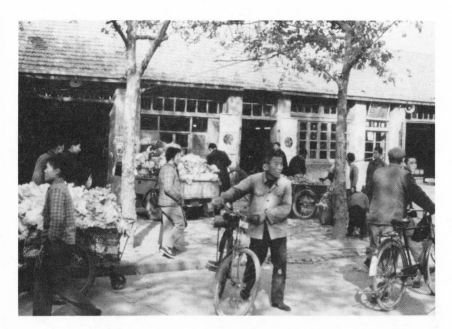

Shopping at Fruit Lake.

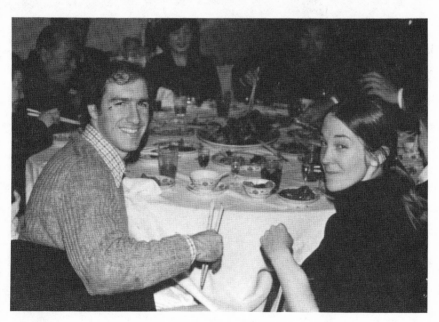

The authors at a banquet shortly after arrival in China.

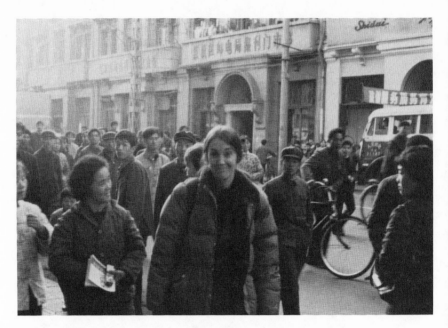

Gail, with Jessie on her back, strolls through Wuhan.

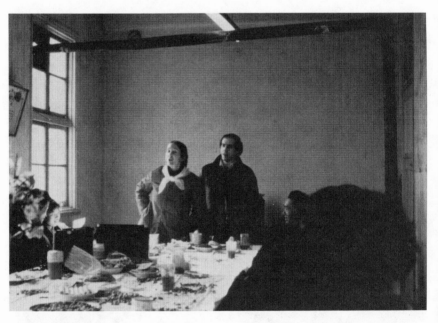

The authors entertain at an English department party. The pipe overhead allows escape of fumes from a coal stove.

3

The Individual and the Institution

As we saw in chapter 2, the ordinary activities of daily life take place within the walls of the work unit. In several important ways, however, the unit fails to conform to the rather appealing notion that it is simply an agricultural village transported to a modern urban setting. As many *danwei* staff noted, the unit is not based on family or kinship ties, although those continue to be an important force in their lives. Rather, the work unit has been created and administered by the state to orchestrate more closely life and work in Chinese communities. This chapter describes the relationship between individual unit members and the administrative apparatus with which they must contend.

Recent visitors to China have been consistently struck by the power that work units exercise over their members' lives.[1] Three French scholars who lived in China from 1972 to 1975 have asserted that the *danwei* "gathers together within the control of a single body all the threads of the individual's life; it measures according to its own standards the tastes, habits and behavior of every person; it is the unit and the norm of work, of life, and of thought . . ." (Broyelle, Broyelle, and Tschirhart 1980, 22). According to these observers, the work unit (and through it, the Chinesee Communist party) is an institution with almost unlimited scope and power, and almost no recourse for its individual members. In our experience, institutional con-

---

1. In an October 1979 *New York Times* article, Fox Butterfield quoted a description of a *danwei* by one of the first American students at Beijing University after normalization of relations between the United States and China: "It's like a womb. You can't get away from it." More recently, A. M. Rosenthal, publisher of the *New York Times*, has joined the list of American observers who have remarked on the centrality of the unit for individual Chinese citizens (A. M. Rosenthal 1981).

trol in the *danwei* was both more complex and less inclusive.[2] Two key indicators of institutional control are freedom of membership and organizational scope. To examine the first, we describe the system of assignment to work units both from a historical perspective and as it worked in our hospital unit. Organizational scope can be defined in terms of the separation of the institution and the individual in the sphere of work and also in terms of the structural divisions between public and private life. We take the second approach, describing the balance between public and private life in our unit.

ASSIGNMENT TO A WORK UNIT

During the decade after 1949, problems of urban development and unemployment were exacerbated by the migration of millions of peasants into the cities. Beginning in the early fifties, the government addressed this problem through a series of regulations that gradually established state control over both the urban and rural population. In the area of work, all enterprises and businesses were socialized, that is, brought under state or collective control and ownership. Thus, labor allocation was eventually centralized and work organizations (*danwei*) were placed under government administration.

In the years 1951–1958, a variety of regulations established a system of household registration that cemented state control over population movement. These regulations included explicit migration rules. Grain-rationing measures for cities and towns were based on household registration of the residents. The registration system was placed under the charge of the public security organization and their local representatives, the residence committees. The residence committees were responsible for health, sanitation, dispute mediation, and public security work for 100 to 600 households, and they were further divided into residence groups of 15 to 40 households (Schurmann 1966). The household registration rules required all citizens to report any change in residence, additions to or deaths in the family, and temporary absences from or visitors to one's home. Regarding migration to the cities, the regulations stated:

> A citizen who wants to move from the countryside to a city must possess a certificate of employment issued by the labor department of the

2. Part of the difference between our interpretation and that of Broyelle, Broyelle, and Tschirhart may be related to changes in the institution observed and in the position of foreigners in China between 1972–1975 (the end of the Cultural Revolution) and 1979–1980 (the moderate aftermath).

city, a certificate of selection issued by a school, or a certificate issued by the household registration organ of the city permitting the removal to the city. (Tien 1973, 380)

Although these regulations did not immediately end the influx of peasants to China's cities, they did reinforce a system of planned labor allocation that eventually slowed the tide.[3] Under this system, initial assignment of jobs and transfers from one work unit to another had to be approved by the labor bureaus and the work units involved. Although abuses of the system have never been eliminated,[4] the following description by a Hong Kong refugee illustrates the degree of control exercised by the state.

"You just can't go out and look for a job in the city because these jobs are carefully parceled out, even the lowest such as street cleaners, transport workers, or toilet cleaners. Almost every unit has to hire its workers through the provincial revolutionary committee [the Cultural Revolution form of government]. The committee decides how many workers can be hired in Fuzhou [a city] acting in accordance with nationally determined quotas. If the central level says "no more jobs," then we can't hire a single person in the city. The central level also imposes harsh restrictions for any urban jobs that are available. . . ." (Frolic 1980, 137)

A second mechanism directed at the problem of urban unemployment dealt specifically with unemployment among urban youth. This was an issue all during the fifties, and in 1957 it was suggested that the youth unable to find jobs or to continue their education in the cities might go to the villages for employment. The intense mobilization of labor power during the Great Leap Forward (1958–1961) interrupted implementation of this idea. Afterward, however, China's leaders confronted the dual dilemma of shrinking urban job opportunities and a rising urban birthrate. The result was the massive resettlement of urban youth known as "Up to the Mountains and Down to the Villages."[5] The program began slowly, transferring over a million graduates of secondary schools between 1962 and 1966. After the start of the Cultural Revolution, which placed great emphasis on the ideo-

3. See Bernstein (1977, 34). In 1954, of 2.45 million urban persons hired, more than two-thirds were peasants. In 1956, one-third of the 2.24 million persons hired were peasants.
4. See Frolic (1980) for a wide variety of descriptions of "going in the back door" for favors, jobs, and the like.
5. This summary is based on Bernstein (1977).

logical reeducation inherent in such a program, virtually all middle school graduates were required to relocate for at least two years.[6] From 1968 to 1978, 17 million urban youth were "sent down" to the countryside. In the mid-seventies, shortcomings in the program were criticized and attempts made to develop policies that would improve living and working conditions for these youth.[7] In addition, many young people were allowed to return to their homes; others simply left the countryside and returned illegally. Although resettlement continues, the regime is now emphasizing more urban job opportunities as a solution to China's rising unemployment among young people.

Thus the characteristics of assignment to a work unit in China have varied during the past thirty years. At first, individual initiative was fairly important, for the state only gradually gained control over rural migration and urban household residence. Following that, an orderly system was established that appeared to place strict limits on the individual's choice of employment. Most rural youth simply stayed on the farm, joining the work team in which they were raised or marrying into a neighboring team. Urban youth were assigned by the labor offices to jobs in the state or collective sectors, or they were sent down to the countryside for an unspecified period. Those fortunate enough to quality for further education were assigned to appropriate positions after graduation. During the Cultural Revolution, this orderly process was disrupted as many more youth from the cities were sent to the countryside and political criteria became more salient in job assignment. Individual career goals, though never the major criteria of job assignment, were completely ignored as massive numbers of youth and older personnel were shipped off to the countryside for reeducation.

Since the Cultural Revolution, with the introduction of more flexible economic policies and the emergence of diverse enterprise arrangements in China's cities, possibilities for the assignment of youth have proliferated and probably also increased their sense of having options. As in the past, rural youth have fewer choices than do urban youth. Unless they qualify for further education, graduates of rural secondary schools (ten million in 1979) go home to work on the land. To counter increasing rural unemployment, the

6. The regulations for exemption from being sent down seem to have varied by time and place. Young people were exempted for reasons of a child's or parent's health. In addition, it seems that one child in each family was not required to go, so an only child and a child whose siblings had gone could stay in the city, although to do so was no guarantee of an urban job assignment (Bernstein 1977, 336, n. 2).

7. These new policies include settling youth together in farms nearer their homes and giving them larger incomes and large "resettlement gifts" (Frolic 1980, 42–57).

government plans to diversify the rural economy (Wei 1980, 21). The approximately three million urban middle school graduates who do not qualify for further education may be assigned to highly prized jobs in urban areas as workers in state or collectively run enterprises or in commercial or government institutions. For the child of a retiring worker, technician, or administrative cadre, the recently promulgated regulation known as *dingti* ("replacement") has established a system of occupational inheritance. Under these rules, a parent retiring from a job in the state sector may pass that job on to a son or daughter.[8] The regime has also encouraged a certain degree of individual initiative in job seeking as it faces the task of assigning both urban middle school graduates and the large number of "sent-down" youth who have now returned to the cities. Many young people have been encouraged to join recently established collectively owned service and small commercial enterprises. In the fall of 1980, the government approved some fifty thousand applications for the creation of free-enterprise businesses such as restaurants, vending booths, and repair shops (Butterfield 1981b). There are plans to reorganize further the program of sending youth to the countryside, to make it more effective *and* appealing (Wei 1980, 16). For graduates of middle schools who must wait months or years to get a job, there are temporary "labor service companies" with teams performing work in construction, service, or repair.[9]

8. For the official regulations on *dingti*, see *Shehui Wenjiao Xingzheng Caiwu Zhidu Zhaibian* (1979, 434). According to Shirk (1981), the *dingti* regulations guarantee a job to one child of every retiring state employee, including workers, technicians, and administrative cadres but not temporary workers or workers in collective enterprises. The candidate must be a graduate of lower middle school, under thirty, and not employed in a state enterprise. See also descriptions of *dingti* in Gold (1980) and Davis-Friedmann (1981).

9. Perhaps more important than these diverse avenues developed to provide jobs for city residents *in* the cities have been policy statements recognizing a need for more flexibility in the overall labor allocation system. In February 1980, for example, the director of the provincial Bureau of Labor announced "a major reform in our system of recruiting workers. In the past, workers were assigned to enterprises by state labor departments under a unified plan. The enterprises had no choice of personnel and could not get all those who were qualified and willing to work there, neither could job-seeking youths choose the jobs or the units they liked. We are changing this system of recruitment. Now those waiting for work can voluntarily apply for jobs and the enterprises or departments concerned can choose the best qualified first through examinations. Both sides have a choice, thereby helping to eliminate the above-mentioned shortcomings. . . . Those who have failed the examinations . . . will be *assigned* appropriate jobs later by state labor departments" (Wei 1980, 15–16; emphasis added).

These reforms, if implemented, promise a potential increase in the system's flexibility and responsiveness to personal desires. In particular, the assignment of recent middle school graduates on the basis of examinations and voluntary applications is a significant step. The role of the Bureau of Labor remains unclear, however, and for people who do poorly on examinations its role is probably unchanged. Furthermore, for staff desiring transfer, the necessity of obtaining permission from both units involved remains a major concern.

Finally, a small number of urban and rural middle school graduates are able to continue their education by passing a nationwide examination, reinstituted in 1977. In 1979, 270,000 of 4.6 million students (5.8 percent) passed the examination (*Beijing Review* 22, no. 41 [12 October 1979]: 6). Students at national-level institutions are drawn from all parts of China, and after graduation are assigned to posts in their home province or in another location. Students accepted to provincial or lower-level schools are generally drawn from that region and assigned to the same area after graduation. The graduates submit a list of preferred locations based on a list of possible job openings, but the final choice is made by the bureaus of labor and education.[10]

ASSIGNMENT TO OUR UNIT

In the hospital and the associated medical college, personnel are divided into three broad occupational categories: cadres (*ganbu*), technicians (*jishuyuan*), and workers (*gongren*). These general categories cover a variety of occupations, each with its own ranking system and wage scale.[11] Administrative and professional personnel in such state-run enterprises are called cadres. In the hospital these include the physicians, the nurses, and the entire range of administrators from the director to the secretaries and assistants. In the medical college, physicians, scientists, teachers, accountants, and administrative personnel are all referred to as cadres. The second category includes the rather small number of medical technicians working in the laboratories in both the hospital and medical college. The third category, workers, encompasses a variety of skilled and unskilled occupations, including cooks, electricians, health aides, plumbers, carpenters, mechanics, laundry people,

10. The recent reevaluation of the importance of intellectuals in the modernization drive has spurred suggestions to "take concrete measures to give full play to the role of intellectuals" (Hu 1981, 16). Among these measures is the proposed reform of the recruitment and promotion of intellectuals: "It is necessary to set up and perfect the system of selecting, checking, promoting, and transferring personnel, a system which would encourage competition. Organs such as talent recruitment or employment offices can be set up, so that all able and talented personnel will be put to good use and given jobs according to ability. In this way, talented personnel, heretofore "owned by the units to which they belong," can work elsewhere and can better develop their talents" (ibid.). These radical reforms, if implemented, would substantially alter the power of the state and the local-level institutions over individual staff members. Given the entrenched position of the units and their leadership, it is difficult to envision such dramatic change except in the highest echelons of intellectual endeavor.

11. For a detailed presentation of the wage system in China, see Korzec and Whyte (1981, 250). For a description of occupational categories in a technical unit, see Blecher and White (1980, 12).

night watchmen, construction workers, and general unskilled workers doing manual labor. The wage scales for various hospital ward personnel are discussed in detail in chapter 4.

The assignment of all staff is handled by several different administrative bodies, depending on the type of job, and the staff appear to be recruited from a variety of labor markets. Medical and technical personnel with advanced training are assigned by the provincial Bureau of Education in conjunction with the Bureau of Labor. Many, especially those assigned before the Cultural Revolution, are from other cities, including Beijing, Shanghai, and Guangzhou. On the other hand, the nurses, low-level technicians, and workers are generally from Hubei, though not necessarily from Wuhan. The workers seem to be the most parochial, with many recruited from the neighborhoods surrounding the hospital. In addition, several workers have replaced their retired parents in the unit, through *dingti*.[12]

The primary characteristic of the staff population in the *danwei* seems to be continuity. Yet important changes in the recruitment of staff have created "generational" differences between staff members and changes in the work unit over time. Most of the older hospital or medical college staff whom we met had lived and worked in their unit for a long time. For example, of the six infectious disease physicians, all of whom were in their forties or fifties, three had worked at the hospital since graduation from medical school twenty to thirty years earlier. Two had been transferred from the other hospital attached to Hubei Provincial Medical College in Wuhan, four and ten years before. One had been transferred three years earlier from a county hospital in the same province. Most of the older teachers and researchers we knew at the medical college had also been assigned to the unit ten or more years before. Finally, the various workers with whom we had contact—two cooks, a mechanic, a laundry person, several day-care workers, and a night watchman—had all lived in the unit since before the Cultural Revolution. The older members of the unit thus represented a fairly stable population, although many of the professional and administrative staff had been recruited from areas outside the city and even the province.

The younger staff, on the other hand, exemplified changes in the assignment system and in the politics of China since 1966. The majority of the staff between ages twenty-five and thirty-five were not assigned directly to

12. *Dingti* is a popular avenue of assignment. Down the road from the hospital is a factory employing 8,000 workers; 200 new workers were assigned through this process in 1979. Unfortunately, it is not known what proportion of all new workers hired in 1979 obtained their assignments through *dingti*.

our *danwei* but, in accordance with Cultural Revolution reforms, had first been sent down to the countryside for further education. Researchers and teachers were admitted to universities after recommendation by their countryside leaders on the basis of political rather than professional criteria. Performance and subsequent assignment to our unit by provincial bureaus were also subject to ideological evaluation. During the Cultural Revolution, nurses, low-level technicians, and workers were recruited ad hoc from both urban and rural areas, but recommendation was also based on radical political criteria.

After the Cultural Revolution and the reversal of the ultra-egalitarian assignment policies, urban children started coming home. The recent innovations to provide more jobs for city residents have thus produced a third "generation" in the *danwei*. Many of the newest members have been assigned directly to the unit either from unit families or from nearby units. Although some children are still required to go to the countryside after graduation, and job assignment through examination has been revived, the emphasis on trying to assign unit members' children close to home seems to be very strong (Shirk 1981), not only for workers but also for professionals. For example, four of the five newest members of the medical college English department, all graduates of the local teachers' college, are the children of health or medical college cadres in Wuhan. Two grew up in our unit, and both are children of medical college administrators. The third is a child of a high-level leader of another medical college. The fourth is from Wuhan, with one parent a former Bureau of Health official. The fifth is from Beijing and hopes to be able to return there to work someday. The recent assignment of technical staff on the basis of qualifying examinations appears to exhibit the same trend. For example, the child of two medical college researchers, previously assigned as a worker in the hospital emergency room, had just passed the examination and been assigned to work as a technician in the medical college. Finally, workers are being assigned close to home as a result of *dingti* and an apparent policy of assigning children to units near their parents' as often as possible. For example, four of our neighbors had at least one child working at the large machine-tools factory down the street, and the eldest daughter of another neighbor had just been assigned to work as a sales clerk in a food store located in the factory unit.

In conclusion, assignment to a work unit is a decision always made by the state. Assignment policies have, however, passed through several stages, and in the process three "generations" have been created within the *danwei*. Each appears to have different histories, friendships, and professional ties, which in turn may lead to a different pattern of dependency on the work unit. The older staff have been in the unit the longest, yet have the most diverse origins and experience. Their personal backgrounds thus provide them with important outside ties that counteract the dependency inherent in longtime unit membership. Those assigned to the work unit during the Cultural Revolution may be the least dependent. Their experience before assignment was highly politicized, and their ties outside the unit are based on ideological rather than occupational bonds. On the other hand, the dramatic eradication of the Cultural Revolution reforms has created a sense of inadequacy among many of these members who are now focusing on the task of "catching up." The third group may be the most dependent on the *danwei*, for their experience outside the unit is the most limited. Their geographic range is the smallest; many have grown up in or near the unit. For these youngest members, the unit most closely resembles an urban village.

LEAVING THE UNIT

Our description so far has emphasized the stability and continuity of life in the *danwei*. Yet there is also a degree of fluidity and flexibility in the system that undoubtedly contributes to its survival. It is not impossible to leave the unit.

Most of our discussion here deals with "exit" (Hirschman 1970) resulting from individual initiative, that is, voluntary departure from the unit. Yet involuntary exit (through transfer) is also a fact of life in Chinese units. For example, one researcher in the medical college was *twice* required to practice different medical specialties for which he was not trained. He was understandably frustrated but said, "What could I do? I accepted it." Incorrect or illogical assignment of personnel is probably an inevitable by-product of a state system of labor allocation in a nation the size of China. Certainly information gathered from refugees in Hong Kong abounds with stories of personal frustration in the face of bureaucratic shuffling of job assignments and reassignments (Bernstein 1977, Frolic 1980).

On the other hand, *danwei* personnel are able to initiate both transfers and unofficial leaves, though not without the resistance of the weight of a bureaucratic system and the vested interest the work units maintain in their staff. An official transfer is the most difficult and time-consuming exit to accomplish. The wife of one member of the medical college staff, for example, waited ten years before being transferred from a city in northern China to work in our unit. A person who wants to change jobs must obtain approval from the leaders of both *danwei* involved, and there must be an opening at the unit to which he or she wants to transfer. In this sense, the criticism that units "own" their staff is justified. For example, the opening of a new hospital in Wuhan resulted in many transfer applications by physicians throughout the province, including several from an older hospital in Wuhan. One such application was approved by the new hospital administrators but denied by those in the older hospital, who did not want to lose the physician's skills. Furthermore, they were worried that if he left the *danwei* it would also be more difficult to keep his wife, a valued medical specialist, from applying for transfer. Thus, transfers based on an individual's personal desire to advance may come into direct conflict with the needs of the institution as perceived by the *danwei* leaders.

However, the individual has some leverage. First, in job assignment and transfer, personal and family constraints—as distinct from personal ambition—are generally given weight. Except during the Cultural Revolution, keeping marriages and families intact has been viewed as a legitimate priority.[13] Indeed, only two of the work unit personnel we knew had spouses living permanently in another location. One was an old master cook whose wife still lived in the countryside in Anhui Province. The other was an administrative secretary who had recently married a cadre working in a city in another part of the province. The secretary hoped that his new wife would eventually be able to find an opening at either our *danwei* or a nearby work unit. The fact that so many spouses worked together in our *danwei* is silent testimony to the importance of the family in job allocation, even if it takes some time to work out the assignments.[14]

As an alternative, a staff member may negotiate some type of nonpermanent exit from a work unit. Such measures include unofficial loaning of staff members to other *danwei*, going to another institution for further study or advanced work experience, and, more recently, going abroad. In this way, staff may invest in their personal careers without threatening the unit.[15] In fact any investment that creates a more valuable staff member makes that person more desirable to the *danwei*. Consequently, most work units encourage their members to pursue further education as long as it

13. See chap. 2, n. 4.

14. Exceptions are family members who live in the countryside and have agricultural household residence. As described above, transfer from the countryside to the city is difficult or impossible.

15. Sending staff to other units does increase horizontal ties between units, which seem to be generally lacking. These connections can produce useful information, potential contacts, help secure supplies, or aid in administration work.

does not interfere with their work. Generally it is the better-educated, professional staff who are in a position to negotiate such a move. However, the recent modernization drive has created an atmosphere in which all staff are encouraged to study and "catch up" (see chapter 4).

Third, in the case of leaders and intellectuals who were the targets of extreme attack during the Cultural Revolution, an attempt has been made to transfer them permanently to other *danwei*. For example, a former medical college official who had been physically attacked and made to walk around for months with a wooden sign around his neck was transferred to head another medical college in the same city immediately after the Cultural Revolution. The rationale was that it would be too difficult for him to function effectively within his old *danwei*. This kind of transfer, however, was usually reserved for the most extreme cases. In our unit, many intellectuals were still forced to deal with their former tormentors daily.[16] Recollection of Cultural Revolution conflicts, and the anger and frustration felt by many now aging intellectuals about their ruined careers can be a major problem for administrators. The script and some of the power positions may have changed, but most of the actors are the same. This situation clearly exacerbates tensions, which may surface in other areas. Thus, it is especially helpful that many of these intellectuals are now receiving further training and are more frequently allowed to leave the *danwei* to advance their careers.

Another way to leave our *danwei* constitutes part of the ordinary work assignment in a hospital unit: rotation to the countryside for teaching, prevention, epidemic, and other medical work. This form of exit is not the result of personal initiative; in fact it is very difficult to avoid. Nevertheless, it provides significant contact with other *danwei* and colleagues not associated directly with our work unit. It also may serve as a kind of safety valve for tensions and frustrations that accumulate within the unit walls.

Sending health professionals to the countryside began in the early fifties, during the major health campaigns carried out by the Ministry of Health. Several doctors in our unit recalled going to the countryside to inoculate peasants against smallpox (1950) and to diagnose and treat syphilis (1953). The massive campaign to eradicate the "four pests" (flies, mosquitoes, rats, and sparrows) in 1958 brought out all medical school students and teachers. For three to four months, volunteer medical personnel worked on the campaign, with special emphasis on detecting schistosomiasis. One doc-

16. See the play by Xing Yixun, *Power versus Law*, translated in *Chinese Literature* 6 (June 1980): 131–91, for an eloquent description of the persistence of Cultural Revolution tensions in a unit.

tor said he went into peasant homes and outhouses to check stools for parasites. From 1958 to 1965, doctors and nurses continued to go to the countryside in rotating medical teams. With the onset of the Cultural Revolution, however, all the staff at both the medical college and the hospital were caught up in struggles and political movements. Many joined mobile medical teams. In 1969 all the teachers, administrators, and medical staff of the college were forced to go to the countryside for ten months, without their families, to engage in political reeducation. The hospital staff continued to rotate down in large numbers.

During the seventies, as political stability returned, approximately one-third of the hospital staff were required to be in the countryside at any given time (Dimond 1971, 1555). Medical college staff were asked less frequently to participate, unless their specialty was directly related to a particular medical problem. (Anatomists, for example, were sent less often than parasitologists.) In the late seventies the program was cut back so that now only 10 percent of hospital staff rotate at a time. Furthermore, instead of going to communes or brigades, the physicians and nurses concentrate on the county hospitals, where they practice medicine, conduct workshops, and teach advanced courses in medical specialties. (The county hospitals are now considered sophisticated enough to assume supervision of commune and brigade medical training, at least in Hubei Province.) This 10 percent includes not only medical personnel going to rural counties, but also those assigned to visit factory clinics, street clinics, and medical missions to foreign nations.

Each of the seventy-two counties in Hubei Province is assigned to one of the national, provincial, or municipal hospitals in Wuhan for purposes of patient referral (see chapter 6) and "mutual exchange." This exchange consists mainly in the temporary assignment of staff from higher-level hospitals to the counties. Our hospital has fifteen assigned counties. Department heads assign their staff for two to six months in rural areas, and each staff member goes every three or four years. Research teams from the hospital and medical college are also dispatched, as well as emergency medical teams in the case of epidemics or difficult medical problems. Repeated visits by the same physicians or nurses establish personal relationships that can make the assignment a positive experience. For example, a husband and wife who had previously worked at a county hospital were generally assigned to that hospital during their rotations. The director of the county hospital was a medical school classmate, and both looked forward to working with him and renewing old ties.

It is difficult to estimate how many people actually leave their *danwei*. Unofficial leaves, foreign-language study, and countryside rotation seem to be much more common than official transfer. Physicians, teachers, and high-level administrators appear to have greater interunit mobility than workers and low-level staff members, primarily because the opportunities and demand for these professionals are greater than for ordinary workers.[17] Leaving the *danwei* permanently, however, is not the norm.

FREEDOM OF MEMBERSHIP

Compared to getting a job in the United States, this system of planned allocation of labor is rigid and authoritarian, taking most of the decision-making power out of the hands of the individual. Indeed, two China scholars have asserted that "generally speaking, individual desires and interests seemed to play little role in this sorting process [of people for jobs]" (Whyte and Parish 1983, 40). Several examples from our unit confirm this observation. Furthermore, although the rationale for the impersonal decision making is ostensibly to create a more equitable system of job distribution, in fact the system is far from impartial. As noted above, except during the height of the Cultural Revolution, urban residents and their children continue to be favored for the better-paying jobs, and those in positions of power often try to influence placement of their children.

For the ordinary Chinese citizen, then, job assignment and transfer are seldom products of individual initiative. In fact individual initiative may instead reflect abuse of the system. The state controls assignment, and the transfer of personnel is under the jurisdiction of the *danwei*. On the other hand, our observations indicate that the wishes of individual staff members are not entirely ignored. Spouses are assigned together, and at least one child in a family generally remains near the parents. Furthermore, although transfer is sometimes difficult, people in our *danwei* definitely viewed it as a viable employment alternative. Unofficial exits from the unit provide an additional way for individuals to meet their needs within the system. Finally, it appears that the recent increase in options for young urban residents may lead to greater responsiveness to individual needs.

The sheer numbers and logistics involved in such a system necessarily

17. There are exceptions, of course. A cook from our unit was assigned to accompany the Hubei medical mission to Algeria for three years. It was, however, the first time he had left Wuhan in fifty-eight years.

limit the strategies that individuals can employ. Furthermore, in this paternalistic system the leadership rather than the individual makes the decisions. During our visit the medical college was allowed to send one candidate to take an examination for further foreign-language study in Beijing. College officials asked a young party member in the English department to stand aside so that a colleague from Beijing might have the opportunity to return to his home. After some persuasion, the party member agreed to do so, despite personal disappointment. Thus, opportunities are mixed: one person is given a chance at the expense of another. The choice is out of the individual's hands.

PUBLIC AND PRIVATE LIFE

The control of the individual by the institution also extends to private life. Privacy can be defined in terms of the amount of per-capita living space, which affects a person's sense of being on display to his or her neighbors.[18] It can also be viewed as the degree to which personal matters such as housing, choice of spouse, the decision to have children, and various family affairs are subjects of concern to—and approval by—work unit leaders.

Daily life in our *danwei* is typical of small communities anywhere. People do not know all the families who live in the hospital unit, but they generally know their neighbors quite well and at least recognize all the people in their apartment building. Mutual dependence and common problems bring people closer together. A backed-up toilet, howling cats at three in the morning, lost family chickens, the arrival of the Sunday puffed-rice exploding cannon, and news of a local "walk-in" movie are all sources of common concern or excitement. When difficulties arise, neighbors pitch in to help. Gossip spreads quickly and personal affairs are rarely secret for long. Crowded living conditions produce a sense of greater visibility and of public display of some aspects of family life. Peer pressure from neighbors and friends to conform to local norms of behavior is inevitably greater under such conditions. Even foreigners are not immune.

Because we were obviously more visible in Chinese society, public in-

18. At the end of 1978, per-capita living space was reported at 3.6 square meters in 192 Chinese cities, much less than in the countryside (*Beijing Review* 23, no. 6 [11 February 1980]: 7). Figures for 1978 published in *Zhongguo Baike Nianjian 1980* [1980 Chinese yearbook] reported 3.9 square meters per person for Wuhan, 4.6 for Beijing, 4.5 for Shanghai, 3.8 for Guangzhou, 3.5 for Tianjin, and 5.0 for Nanjing.

trusion into our private lives was probably exaggerated. We encountered blatant pressure to change our Western child-rearing habits. At first our friends tried to be discreet. Seeing our daughter with a plastic bottle in her mouth, they assumed that her mother had no milk. Seeing her severe diaper rash when we sought medical attention, they gently advised Chinese open-air trousers. Strong opposition finally surfaced on the issue of where Jessie slept at night. The unacceptability of her being in a room alone was made clear to us not only by her day-care teacher, but also by our neighbors and the nursing staff of the infectious disease ward. We accepted this criticism with grace, and Jessie moved into our bedroom.

In more subtle ways, the public display of private life is increased by the physical structure of the *danwei* housing. The master cook assigned to us for the first two months came to work in our apartment three times a day. The kitchen had several windows, which were often open to ventilate the coal fumes. The cook was a gregarious fellow and a longtime resident of the hospital unit. Consequently, his sojourn with foreigners was not surprisingly a subject of general interest and discussion. Each day he would stand at our second-floor kitchen window, and when acquaintances came by he would talk to them as he cooked. Sometimes it seemed as if the people outside were right in our apartment. It was the same when we did our laundry. Every Sunday morning, one of us would scrub the week's clothes on a small washboard in the kitchen sink. Children playing outside the window would watch us and comment on our efforts. Friends passing by would say hello. As we hung up our clothes on the line that stretched across our balcony, we drew comments from passersby. Imperceptibly the way we did our wash began to change, and we were happy when it looked like everyone else's, turned inside out, pants hanging down with pockets flapping.

A neighbor's wedding plans were obvious when his parents began construction of the nuptial bed and wardrobe on their balcony, where neighbors and friends could evaluate the quality and cost. Balconies served as storage closets, chicken coops, plant stands, and places to sit and watch the world go by. Those without balconies sit by the side of the building, alone or with friends. These watchful eyes, in addition to the guard at the unit front gate, prevent any visitors from coming or going unobserved. Young couples trying to catch a few quiet moments find it hard to avoid being seen. In fact anyone doing anything out of the ordinary attracts attention, and once that occurs, anonymity is lost. Although we were not privy to normal patterns of gossip, it seemed that people knew a great deal about each other's lives, certainly about the impact of the Cultural Revolution upon members of the unit and about current events and blooming romances among neighbors and friends.

Aren't people frustrated with so little privacy? Studies of Chinese living in other countries have shown that it is possible to develop coping strategies in conditions of close communal living (E. N. Anderson 1972). Our own observations indicated that people in our unit did not necessarily consider themselves deprived of privacy. First, several people reminded us that the housing conditions in our *danwei* were thought to be better than those in other units and some other cities. Second, and more important, despite the visibility of some aspects of private life, families could and did live behind closed doors. Young people managed to find privacy for courtships and quiet times. Roommates accommodated young lovers, and the parks were full of young couples. Finally, Chinese perceptions of the need for privacy may differ from Western assumptions.[19] For example, when we asked a young teacher who lived with parents, sister, wife, and two-year-old daughter if he wanted to be alone with his wife more, he responded, "I don't want to leave my parents." His concern was time for his studies, not time to be alone.

The implementation of unit regulations by the unit leaders is also a force in the private lives of staff members. Marriage, divorce, childbearing, education, job assignment, job transfer, and the resolution of conflicts all involve the knowledge and, in most cases, approval of these leaders; they are also responsible for the personal well-being of their staff.

First of all, unit leaders control the housing assignment of a staff member when he or she joins the *danwei*. A person who is assigned or transferred to the work unit first applies to the unit housing office, located in the hospital administration building. If no housing is available, the staff member is placed on a waiting list and must seek alternatives such as living with relatives or obtaining housing (not necessarily near the hospital) through a management office that distributes housing in urban neighborhoods. Construction of two new apartment buildings during our visit did much to alleviate the housing shortage in our unit.

As staff members' housing requirements change over the years—as families expand, children grow up, and grandchildren arrive—the unit housing office is responsible for assigning housing appropriate to these needs. According to Broyelle, Broyelle, and Tschirhart, "the power which [the leadership] exercises in these matters can become only too easily a

19. See Munro (1979) for a discussion of the differences between Western and Chinese views on the private realm of the self.

weapon which can be turned against its employees" (1980, 26). There is little doubt that this was the case during the Cultural Revolution, when those who made political errors were deprived of housing benefits. Many of these abuses, however, have now been reversed. Although we had little opportunity to observe the inner workings of the *danwei's* housing office, the allocation of the newly constructed apartments appeared to be based on rational criteria; those who had waited the longest, had the most pressing need for more space, or had been wronged during the Cultural Revolution were given priority. Whyte and Parish conclude that "With such a cramped housing supply and allocation through slow-moving bureaucratic channels, the rate of residential mobility within Chinese cities has remained low." (1983, 81). Members of *danwei*, with access to their own housing office, may have a slightly easier time than urbanites who must deal with an impersonal city housing authority.

Marriage is another area in which unit leaders potentially exercise a great deal of control. Officially, marriages must be registered and approved in the government marriage registration office. This office, however, apparently relies almost entirely on approval by the couple's respective *danwei* leaders. Those without such approval will not be registered for marriage. Approval is generally forthcoming except when the people are considered too young, or when one is in some way politically suspect.[20] Yet even as a passive form of control, this represents an important power that the institution can exercise over its members.

When a couple is ready to have children, the state, acting through the local work (or neighborhood) small group, also plays an important role. National family planning policies recommending one or two children per couple are reinforced at the local level by strong economic incentives. Those who promise to have only one child are rewarded with the housing space allocated for two children, and the child is given free day care, education, medical care, and other benefits. Those choosing to have more than two children are penalized by a loss in similar benefits for the third child. The campaign to limit families to one child was just getting underway during our visit. In the hospital, the first hundred women who volunteered for sterilization after one child were rewarded with a substantial cash bonus, and a special ward was set up for them as they recuperated from their sur-

20. Whyte and Parish (1983). Apparently unit leaders are involved in such decisions only when an applicant would clearly have something to lose by marrying a politically backward or criminal individual—as in the case of a party member or a person with a high-level or sensitive position.

gery. Several nurses and a neighbor who got married during this time joined in the campaign by promising to have only one child—without undergoing actual sterilization—and received additional benefits from their work units. Many units, such as the factory down the street, keep colorful charts displaying the declining fertility of their female staff. One woman who became pregnant with her third child was persuaded by her work leaders to have an abortion. We did not observe outright public enforcement of the family planning policies.[21] When it does occur, the unit conducts public criticism meetings. In an extreme case that we were told had occurred several years before, a young, unmarried nurse became pregnant for the second time. A public meeting was held to criticize her. The moral was made explicit that young people should occupy themselves with socialist development instead of with sexual experiments. The nurse obtained an abortion, found it difficult to continue working under this stigma, and was subsequently transferred to a different medical unit.

The mediation of disputes and the enforcement of legal and social norms are also under the jurisdiction of the *danwei* leadership.[22] In urban neighborhoods not attached to production units, these functions are carried out by the residence committees and groups, in conjunction with the public security bureau. Our observations indicate that in work units like ours the residence committees have a negligible role. We did observe old women mobilized by the committees sweeping the sidewalks. However, many of the functions and services of a neighborhood committee appear to be carried out by the unit and the unit leadership. Furthermore, staff who do not live in the unit are still monitored by the unit leaders, and by a residence committee or by another unit where they live. We were told that when personal conflicts or problems in a family occur, such as a child getting into trouble with the police or a married couple quarreling, a leader who is close to the people may become involved. Mediation by local leaders or responsible neighbors is also mandatory before a couple desiring a divorce is allowed to go to court.

In summary, the *danwei* system is structured so that the leadership may exercise a great deal of power over the staff. At the very least, the regula-

21. More commonly it takes the forms of prevention and monitoring female reproductive cycles within work groups (Martin K. Whyte, personal communication).

22. Informal dispute mediation in China is a traditional method of resolving problems under local jurisdiction. The role of the residence committees as the first mediator, prior to formal legal intervention, is thus not an innovation of the current regime. See van der Sprenkel (1962) for a description of a dispute settlement in imperial China, and Lubman (1967) for details on dispute resolution in Chinese neighborhood organizations after 1949.

tions concerning various areas of private life exist as a passive form of control. In chapter 5 we will examine the strategies employed by *danwei* members to offset this control. At this point we must conclude that the concentration of control over private life, reinforced by the conditions of daily living described above and in chapter 2, is profound.

INSTITUTIONAL CONTROL

The degree of *danwei* control over staff, and of staff dependence on the work unit, varies according to a number of factors. These include the member's age, occupation, location of housing (inside or outside the *danwei*, with or without spouse and family), length of association with the *danwei*, nature and extent of outside ties, political history, and party membership. The interrelationship of these variables creates a complex pattern of institutional control.

Although daily routines are conducted within work unit walls, intensifying a sense of community and the force of peer pressure to conform to the norms of life, the *danwei* does not control contact with people outside the unit. People leave the *danwei* every day. Staff may live elsewhere. Family may work in another unit. People visit relatives on Sundays and holidays. Children are assigned to another part of the city or to the countryside. Staff members themselves secure transfers, unofficial leaves, or rotate to the countryside. A few go to Algeria or even the United States.

The leaders in Chinese work units have more involvement in and influence on the daily life and decisions of the ordinary Chinese citizen than is the case in many other countries. In part, this circumstance arises from the bureaucratic allocation of goods, jobs, housing, and other commodities under a planned, socialist regime. In addition, the regime has consciously established a system wherein the local-level leadership (in the person of the *danwei* leader) is responsible for enforcing certain policies, such as family planning, late marriage, and observance of public safety, all of which unquestionably place a great deal of potential power in the hands of the local official. For work unit members there are few options available in housing, education, employment, family size, and even in what to buy at the market. Presumably, this lack of alternatives increases the dependence of unit members on the institution (Stinchcombe 1970). The leaders—and through them, the work unit—clearly have an entrée into an individual's private life. Yet unless the individual transgresses against the regime, control often remains passive.

Recent observers of China are correct in singling out the work unit as a chief element of institutional control over Chinese citizens. The nature of life in a *danwei* facilitates such control. It is easy to know just what is going on with one's neighbors and workmates and difficult not to be affected by what they think and do. It is easy for a work leader to become involved with the private lives of his or her staff when they are neighbors, and it is probably difficult for them to object to this involvement when so much of their lives is dependent on the *danwei* and its leaders. It is a unique environment, and the elements of social control are immediately apparent. Yet the less obvious elements of individual options and changes over time also play a role. Furthermore, an outsider's impressions may distort the reality as perceived by those within the work unit walls. The control of the unit leadership over decisions such as marriage, childbearing, and divorce may not be perceived as all-encompassing if it is rarely exercised, or if the underlying policies find support among unit members. Crowded living conditions and neighborly involvement in daily life may mean lack of privacy to Westerners but not to those living in the unit. In fact, living in such units, where life and work are long-standing commitments, may ease the loneliness and normlessness experienced by many Western urbanites in their modern, free cities.

4

Working in the *Danwei*: The Infectious Disease Ward

THE SETTING

The infectious disease (ID) ward occupies one wing of the first floor of the hospital. To reach the ward, one enters the main door of the hospital, moving through a foyer and into the main hallway. The outside doors to the hospital are open during the day. At night all but one are closed and locked. In the winter, the open doorway is covered by a black cotton padded material to keep out the wind and the bitter cold. Lifting up this heavy swinging door is an awkward and difficult maneuver. Depending on the weather, the floor is either muddy or dusty, gray with dirt from the shoes, bicycles, and carts moved in and out each day. The walls are institutional green, with peeling paint. There is a bust of Mao opposite the doorway, though it may have been removed since we left. On either side of this bust are display cases for political propaganda pictures. Like the glass cases on either side of the circular driveway, these often contain nationally distributed pictures: photographs of criminals on trial in Shanghai or of the Chinese Communist party chairman planting trees to commemorate some holiday. One case is devoted to hospital news, featuring such items as a new austerity campaign or the list of running champions at a local race. On the right as one enters is a little pharmacy, restocked three times a week from larger hospital stores. To the left is a door leading to the electrocardiogram room. Across the hallway is a small window. Behind this three or four women and their abacuses are kept busy accounting for the hospital's debits and credits.

The hospital is laid out like a giant, three-story X, with a library providing a small fourth-story cap. The legs of the X are the hospital wards; at their intersection are a double staircase, auxiliary offices for radiology and

47

laboratory tests, and a small pharmaceutical factory. Administrative offices are in a separate building. The hallway leading to the infectious disease ward is crowded with staff-owned bicycles, all locked and jammed together along the wall. The smells are pungent, an unforgettable mixture of burning coal from the hospital boiler room, formaldehyde, and, occasionally steam rising from the radiators, combined with the odor of human excrement as one passes a much-used public bathroom. The hall is narrow and crowded. One often runs into health aides pulling metal carts used to deliver food to patients, or into the nurses pulling the hospital carts piled high with laundry, clean sheets and white coats. Patients' family members pack this hall as they wait to cook meals for their sick relatives at the tiny kitchen provided for this purpose next to the boiler room.

At the end of this hall, the neurology ward is to the left, and the infectious ward is located farther along on the right. This back hallway is wide and dark and silent. A crack of light shines between the locked double doors of the ward (only opened to bring the food cart in and out).[1] Because the infectious disease ward is an isolation ward, only staff and relatives of critically ill patients are allowed in.[2] Before reaching that locked door, one passes the infectious disease laboratory, staffed with one or two technicians. Directly to the left of the laboratory is the single door through which all staff pass to enter the ward. Each member has a key.

Entering the ward (see figure 6), one first comes to the washroom. Here are lockers in which to hang coats, shoes, and other belongings; and a gray sink with hot water, soap, and a pan of disinfectant to soak one's hands. These pans are located all over the ward, and in lieu of rubber gloves, which are rarely available, they are the main method of disinfecting hands. During cold winter days the three-minute soak in the icy solution is a test of endurance. Behind the washroom are a bathroom, shower, and a smaller room in which staff store clothes and shoes worn on the ward.

Past the washroom doorway, one enters the dark, long hall of the ward. When people talk, their voices echo up and down the hall; when staff members want each other, particularly during the bustle of morning rounds, they often just yell. At most other times, the hall is very quiet, perhaps in part because few relatives can visit these potentially contagious pa-

<hr/>

1. Food is served to patients who are on special diets or on wards where relatives are not allowed to come in and care for them. Patients with no dietary restrictions may either order food from the hospital kitchen or their relatives may come in and cook food for them.

2. A 1978 Ministry of Health regulation mandated a separate ward for these patients, who previously had been assigned to internal medicine.

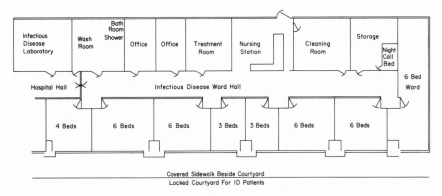

Figure 6. The Infectious Disease Ward

tients. Relatives often line up outside the ward windows in the courtyard to talk to a patient or to peer in and watch. In most wards, relatives
take on many nursing tasks, and the quota of nurses assigned to wards takes
this fact into account.

Patient ward rooms are on the right side of the hall, and staff offices,
nursing station, and various cleaning or storage rooms are on the left. The
floor is gray terrazzo, like all the others, and is kept scrupulously clean,
mopped with disinfectant several times daily. The gray cement extends half-
way up the wall; the top half of the wall is painted white. From the inside
hallway, tall windows look into the patients' ward rooms and the offices.
White cotton curtains, with the name of the hospital in red characters, cover
the lower third of the windows, and patients' activities are easily viewed.

There are eight patient ward rooms, and the patients are separated according to sex, disease, and severity of illness. The first room to the right
has four beds for women with dysentery; the second, six beds for schisto-
somaisis; the third, six beds for men with dysentery and epidemic hemorrhagic fever. The two smaller rooms in the middle of the ward, with three
beds each, are reserved for critically ill patients. Many patients are moved
into these beds before they die. The sixth and seventh ward rooms have six
beds each for males with hepatitis. The last ward room has six beds for female hepatitis patients. Each male ward room shares a bathroom with the
adjoining one. Each female ward has its own bathroom.

The rooms are neat, even spartan. Each patient has a bed, an off-white
hospital quilt with the red character of the hospital's name printed in the
middle, a pillow, a bedside table, a straight-back chair, pans for eating and

washing, and a thermos for boiled water. Ambulatory patients wear their own clothes in bed. Bedridden patients wear blue-and-white striped hospital pajamas with a dark blue knee-length padded cotton robe. In winter the heat in the ward comes on briefly at eight in the morning and eight in the evening. At other times the ward is often chilly, but the quilts and robes are very warm. In summer, when the ward is hot, ceiling fans and crushed ice bring relief. For patients who are able to walk around, there are doors leading from the patient bathrooms to the locked courtyard outside their windows. Patients can come and go as they please and are found strolling in the courtyard, hanging out laundry, or sitting in the sun on a cold day. From each ward, tall, wide windows look out onto the courtyard, and as the ceiling of the ward itself is fifteen feet high, the patient ward rooms have a pleasant airiness.

In the physicians' offices and the treatment room are standard desks and straight-back chairs. The office prepared for our use contains desks painted bright orange, a locked cabinet, a thermos, and hooks behind the door on which to hang our coats. The treatment room contains the equipment for procedures performed on the ward and is used by both nurses and physicians. Next on the left is the nursing station, the center of activity for the ward staff. The nursing station is enclosed on two sides by a four-foot-high terrazzo counter, with shelves underneath, which defines the working area. Here nurses congregate, some physicians write in the charts, and at least one nurse is on duty to answer the phone and watch the patient buzzers. A panel of lights on the wall lights up and sounds when a patient calls for assistance. Often two or three nurses and health aides stand or sit at three desks in the middle of the station. In spare moments they may wind cotton around sticks to make swabs, sharpen needles for reuse, or prepare medicine trays for the patients. The nursing station also contains the patients' charts; the bed chart, which shows location and degree of illness; a cabinet in which contaminated articles are exposed to evaporating formaldehyde; and more basins for hand soaking. Behind the nursing station are the cleaning room, a small boiler that dispenses hot water, and a cot for physicians who are on night duty. In the ceilings of the ward rooms and offices are long, modern fluorescent lights.

All the staff wear the same style white coat and cap, so that it is initially difficult to differentiate the doctors from the nurses, technicians, and health aides. This practice may change as rank levels are gradually reintroduced into these four jobs. During our stay, even the vice-director of the hospital, a senior infectious disease physician, displayed no sign of his rank. Once people start working, however, their roles are easy to differentiate. The head nurse often says, "We are all equal, but there is a division of labor." And true enough, there are highly articulated rules about the tasks required for each job.

THE STAFF

Nurses

The infectious disease ward had nine nurses (*hushi*) and two assistant head nurses (*fuhushizhang*). While we were there, one was promoted to head nurse (*hushizhang*). All the nurses in our hospital are women; those on our ward range in age from twenty-six to the early fifties. Nursing is hard work, and retirement comes earlier than for some other professions. All the nurses on the ward were married (two during our stay in China). It is common for nurses to be married to physicians, as were three on our ward. Other spouses included drivers, mechanics, and industrial workers. The head nurse, assistant head nurse, and two other nurses lived in hospital housing. Before the two newly married nurses moved in with their husbands, they lived in the hospital dormitory for single nurses. Other nurses lived in work units a short bike or bus ride from the hospital. One nurse lived across the city and rode the bus for an hour each day.

Although nurses have a separate wage scale, they are considered cadres (*ganbu*) along with doctors, teachers, scientists, and administrators. At high levels of administration, many cadres are Communist party members. However, on the infectious disease ward only one of the younger nurses and a senior physician were party members. As cadres, the nurses receive medical insurance coverage for themselves and their children (for a small fee)[3] and other benefits, including a retirement salary and holiday and maternity leaves. Their salaries are generally lower than those of other cadres and workers in state-owned enterprises, beginning at about 35–40 yuan per month, and rarely reaching 70–100 yuan. Forty to 50 yuan seems the norm for an experienced nurse. Until recently, hospital staff did not receive bonuses, a fact that further widened the gap between their earnings and those of industrial workers who earn bonuses. However, in the spring of 1980 the

3. Hubei Provincial Medical College maintains an insurance program for cadre staff children at an annual cost of twelve yuan per child. This is a local program, not typical of cadres in other parts of China.

hospital introduced overtime for those willing to work on holidays, thus bringing additional increments in pay.

The Cultural Revolution had a profound impact on the training and performance of all health care professionals. Before 1966 two nursing schools in Hubei Province, the Wuhan Medical College Teaching Hospital (*Wuyi Zhaoxue Yiyuan*) and the Hubei School of Nursing (*Hubei Hushi Xuexiao*), had three-year, Western-style nursing programs. During the Cultural Revolution both nursing schools closed. In 1973 they reopened and offered an abbreviated, two-year program, and nurses began to graduate again in 1975. During the nine years in which no new nurses graduated, women were recruited for hospital work on the basis of recommendations from their local *danwei* or rural production brigade. These women received on-the-job training, and almost no background in basic sciences was required or provided. They began as health aides; upon recommendation by the hospital unit and passing a local examination, they were promoted to the position of nurse. Consequently, nurses' training backgrounds vary in accordance with their ages. On the infectious disease ward, the youngest nurse had graduated from a two-year program, two nurses in their late twenties had been trained on the job, and those in their thirties and forties had received training in three-year institutions.

This situation was further complicated by the Cultural Revolution policy of rearranging job descriptions to eliminate discrimination. In a hospital setting, the new values dictated that doctors, nurses, and health aides all have an opportunity to perform a variety of tasks. Many nurses became practicing physicians, and some continued to practice for a number of years. Likewise, some high-level administrators, physicians, and technical researchers were criticized for elitist attitudes and demoted to menial positions.

After the Cultural Revolution, the return to earlier ideas about the necessity of a division of labor created several problems. Should nurses and other health personnel who had not received formal training in health sciences continue to work in their jobs? If so, how could their technical level be raised to guarantee adequate levels of expertise without their return to school? If not, how could those unfit for their present jobs be weeded out? One of the thorniest problems was the issue of experienced nurses who had been working as physicians for several years, enjoyed their work, and did not want to become nurses again. Finally, what could be done to compensate for the many years lost by experts who had been away from their specialties for so long that competence would be a serious issue?

Meetings took place at all levels for discussion of these issues. The government had directed that schools open before the actual end of the Cultural Revolution, so personnel were being more adequately trained by 1976. After 1976, job categories began to reflect training. According to one of the ward physicians, "Before 1976, everyone was 'comrade' [*tongzhi*] and there were no job categories. We've just started calling people different titles since 1976 or so." After 1976 the government also directed that classes be provided for those who lacked a firm technical foundation so that they could catch up; that exams be given and promotions made so that people with the appropriate training held the correct jobs; and that the division of jobs and job categories gradually return to pre–Cultural Revolution status.

In 1977 nurses on the infectious disease ward and all over the city began attending continuing education classes to prepare for a qualifying and promotional examination in the spring of 1980. In addition to these night classes, one afternoon each week—in our hospital, Friday—was devoted to education. Depending on their experience and career goals, the nurses were divided into two classes, one for nurses who wanted to be physicians or nursing teachers, and one for those who would take a nationwide examination for nursing certification (exempting those who had been nurses for more than twenty years). During the Cultural Revolution, 150 older, experienced nurses from the First and Second Attached Hospitals of Hubei Provincial Medical College, out of a total of approximately 600 nurses, worked as doctors at some time. Their preparation for this examination was rigorous. For each course they attended evening classes twice a week, totaling about forty hours. Upon completion of each course, they took an examination administered by the provincial Bureau of Health. This resolution of an unusual situation was a onetime occurrence. In the future, promotional ladders for nurses and physicians will be completely distinct.

The resolution of this issue was not without difficulties or exceptions. Several nurses became physicians after 1976, and several others were not required to take the examination but were allowed to continue to practice medicine. The case-by-case approach to each individual situation in the hospital reflects both the difficulty of the issue and the extent of the efforts made to take special circumstances into account. Following are several examples of the decisions made.

1. The surgery department has two nurses who became general surgeons during the Cultural Revolution and still practice surgery. They will remain surgeons but will be ineligible for promotions.
2. In 1978, a very industrious and intelligent nurse in the department of internal medicine was offered the opportunity to become a physician. She did a kind

of internship under the supervision of internists in that department and performed quite well. In 1979, however, the administration asked her to give up her goal. She was offered, instead, a supervising position in radiologic testing, which was more technical than professional. She was not enthusiastic about the job but accepted several months later, realizing that her future potential as a physician would be limited because she would probably not be promoted.

3. In 1977, the head nurse of the hospital was allowed to become a doctor. One year later, the administration asked her to become a nurse again. She agreed, apparently because she felt ill-prepared to function as a physician.

4. During the Cultural Revolution, a nurse in gastroenterology became a gastroenterologist. Because she performed well, she will probably remain a physician. She performs primarily endoscopy and sigmoidoscopy, circumscribed procedures.

During our stay, the nurses were preparing for their examinations (see appendix 5 for sample lectures), and new ranking systems awaited these results. While we were on the infectious disease ward, nursing tasks were shared by all nurses, with the head nurses assuming extra responsibility. The nurses continually rotated among three shifts: nursing shift (*huliban*), a treatment shift (*zhiliaoban*), and a chief shift (*zhuban*). Each week, two or three nurses were assigned to the nursing shift and two nurses to the treatment shift. A new nurse was assigned each day to the chief shift. Their duties are summarized below. (For a complete list of nursing duties, see appendixes 1–3.)

Nursing Shift
1. General nursing: In the morning listen carefully at morning report and know which patients are critical. Check wards to see who needs water, change of clothes, and so on. Then do all personal things for critical patients (wash face, brush teeth). Watch for bed sores. Feed serious patients. Tell special nursing about problems of all critical patients. Count all equipment, bedding, and clothes and get clean clothes from laundry.
2. Special nursing: Help general nursing nurse. Assume responsibility for nursing of critical patients. Listen to report of last shift. Report to next shift about special problems of critical patients.

Treatment Shift
1. General treatment: Give shots, intramuscular shots, intravenous (IV) fluids, prepare treatment equipment for next shift, tell next shift about shortages in medicine.
2. Special Treatment: Change tubings, oversee Monday afternoon sterilization of ward, change sterile fluid for needles, watch supply of oxygen. Help in general treatment.

Chief Shift
Make sure physician's orders are carried out by the treatment nurses, and sign the patient's chart when orders are completed. Update patients' medicine cards.

Send orders to the pharmacy, bring medicine from the pharmacy, and give it to the patients. Call outpatient department and report number of empty beds. Show new patients around the ward.

The new system will probably separate people along the following lines. The nurses' aides (*huliyuan*) will be those promoted from health aide (and those nurses who fail to pass the qualifying examination) and will perform nursing shift duties. The nurses (*hushi*) will be graduates from nursing schools and those who pass the examination, and will carry out the treatment and chief shift duties. The nursing teacher (*hushi*) will be promoted from nurse after the examination, and will be responsible for teaching, writing, and difficult work on the wards. In addition to this professional route for nurses, there will also continue to be an administrative route, involving ward head nurses, department head nurses, and high-level administrative positions. As one of the ward nurses commented, "It will be a better system [because] it separates people with more experience from those just arrived."

The shift from egalitarianism to the anticipated gradation of job levels is reflected in trends of address. "Comrade" (*tongzhi*) was the norm during the Cultural Revolution, and all professional titles were eschewed. Gradually, "doctor" (*daifu*), "department chief" (*zhuren*), and other high-level administrative titles have returned in medical settings, as well as in auxiliary occupations; a cook's apprentice is called "apprentice" (*tudi*), and a main cook is called "master" (*shifu*). Among nurses and health aides, the only division that had emerged in 1980 was one between the nurse and the head nurse.

Doctors

There were eleven physicians assigned to the infectious disease ward, although only five or six practiced there during the fall and winter. While we were at Hubei, five physicians regularly attended rounds, four held the title of resident physician (*zhuyuan yisheng*) pending the 1980 promotions, and one had recently been named department head (*zhuren*) of infectious disease. The hospital vice-director (*fuyuanzhang*) was also an infectious disease specialist and by virtue of his position was acknowledged the ultimate authority on the ward. He conducted rounds no more than once a week, however, and left most of the leadership to the department head. Six other doctors assigned to the ward were not present during our stay: one was in the outpatient department's infectious disease section, one was on leave for six months learning English, one was on leave for six months learning Japanese, one had been sent down to the countryside to assist at a county hospital, one had just been sent to a national hospital in Sichuan Province for one year to learn more about the immunology of hepatitis, and one was part of the Hubei Province medical mission to Africa, on a two-year tour of duty in Algeria. In the spring and summer, when infectious diseases are common, several of the physicians on leave for language study or in the countryside would be called back to the ward.

Of the six physicians on the ward at some time while we were there, three were married to other physicians (two working at Hubei, one at the provincial government hospital nearby); two were married to nurses (both working on the ward, although one transferred from the position of head nurse to the less demanding job of day-care "doctor" because of ill health); and one was married to a professor of science at a university across the lake. Four of the six lived in hospital apartments; the other two (both female) lived with spouses in nearby *danwei* and bicycled to work each day.

About half of the physicians on the infectious disease ward are female. The hospital vice-director is male, but the infectious disease department head is female. In terms of this distribution, the infectious disease ward seems typical of internal medicine in general. However, some specialties within internal medicine are highly sex segregated. Females predominate in obstetrics, gynecology, and pediatrics,[4] males in neurology. In contrast to internists, 95 percent of the surgeons are male. One of the few female surgeons, who was a hepatitis patient on the infectious disease ward during our stay, explained the phenomenon. "Surgeons and internists get the same pay, but [surgery is] a more difficult specialty. Women find it especially difficult. The hours are longer and more tiring. Night duty is more common. When I was pregnant with my third child at age thirty-eight, I found it hard to take the schedule, so I decided to specialize in hand surgery— where you can *sit down* while you work."

Physicians, like nurses, are cadres—government staff assigned to practice medicine within the confines of a bureaucratic institution. With few exceptions, private practice is not permitted.[5] Physicians receive a salary from the state, beginning at 50–60 yuan per month and rising to over 100 yuan. A family with two experienced physicians can easily make 150–200 yuan per

4. Participants in a 1973 U.S. medical delegation to China reported that 97 percent of obstetricians and gynecologists and 75 percent of pediatricians are female (Committee on Scholarly Communication with the People's Republic of China 1973, 125 and 155).

5. Foreign Broadcast Information Service, *Daily Report of the People's Republic of China* 9 September 1981, L33), reports that some physicians—"traditional practitioners, licensed practitioners, and retired practitioners providing services in poor, sparsely populated areas"—may engage in private practice. See also chap. 7.

month. Promotions and salary increases were being discussed while we were there, but no decision was reached before we left. The lowest-level physician, the resident physician, received 60 yuan per month. Although salary increases are not always associated with rank promotions, it was expected that some rise would come when the majority of resident physicians were promoted to the next level, attending physician (*zhuzhi yisheng*).

Contrary to popular belief, the Cultural Revolution had a dramatic impact on physicians. Physicians and specialists did not stop performing their jobs entirely, but they took on some duties of other occupations, particularly symbolic tasks such as cleaning or sweeping. Another important characteristic of this period was the general lack of supervision of work. One physician said, "Before 1975, medical records may not be useful. Then people just looked after their own patients. We didn't have general rules or standards for care." Another added, "Between 1966 and 1971 there was no supervision at all. During this time, if someone asked for advice, we gave it, but otherwise no one volunteered any. Before 1972 it was bad. After 1972, some order was restored to the hospital. But it was really 1976 and 1977 that order returned."

The reconstruction of the medical profession parallels that of nursing. All three medical colleges in Wuhan, Wuhan Medical College (*Wuhan Yixueyuan*), Hubei Medical College (*Hubei Yixueyuan*), and Chinese Traditional Medicine College (*Zhongyi Yixueyuan*), reopened in 1973. The three-year curriculum was expanded to five in 1977, and national entrance examinations were reinstituted at that time. A postgraduate program was reestablished in 1979. Continuing education programs reflect an attempt to compensate for deficiencies in the training of physicians enrolled in three-year medical schools during the Cultural Revolution. It is a gigantic task, one that the authorities admit will be impossible to fulfill adequately. Reinstitution of rankings, promotions, qualifying examinations, and a general return to the pre-1966 structure were all taking place while we were at the hospital. Under current plans, the fifth year of a medical school program will be an internship (*shixi yisheng*) at one of the medical school's attached teaching hospitals. When that is completed, medical students will be assigned by the Bureau of Education to a hospital that has positions to fill, and the student will serve as a resident physician for two to four years. Upon passing a state promotion examination, the resident will advance to the position of attending physician.

While we were there, these regulations for the future were made clear, but remained uncertain regarding the examination and promotion of prac-

ticing physicians whose careers had been disrupted by the Cultural Revolution. As with the promotion of nurses, individual circumstances are taken
into account. In the spring of 1980, a token examination in English was
given to all hospital physicians, and the president of the medical college announced that all physicians would have a chance to take leave to study English. After this examination, however, it was decided that the rest of the
promotion examination would be waived for physicians who had been practicing for a number of years and (by consensual agreement) were qualified.
Subsequent meetings were planned to discuss nominations for attending
physician, department chief, or professor of medicine; names would be
submitted to the medical college, and in turn to the province. The only restriction seemed to be a limit on the percentage of physicians recommended, which was set by the provincial Bureau of Health. These meetings
were just beginning when we left. Most of the physicians who expected a
promotion seemed to feel certain that they would get one. After this onetime event, qualifying examinations would be required for promotion from
resident to attending physician; a committee review of work and publications for those desiring to enter academic medicine may also become a
requirement.

During this period of readjustment, the schedule of physicians on the
infectious disease ward resembled that of doctors in private practice more
than it would under normal conditions (see chapter 8). Without student
doctors and interns—members of the new fifth-year class would not reach
that stage in their training until 1982—the physicians simply came to the
ward and took care of the patients assigned to them. Rounds themselves did
not serve as the arena of formal medical training that they were and will be
in the near future. Thus one important aspect of a teaching hospital was un-
available to us in this study.

Health Aides

There were three health aides (*weishengyuan*) assigned to the infectious
disease ward: a middle-aged female, an eighteen-year-old female, and a
seventeen-year-old male. Both of the latter lived with their parents in hospital apartments. All were under the direction of the head nurse on the ward.
In addition to their cleaning duties, they assisted the nurses in any tasks that
needed extra hands. The older health aide was the nominal director of the
younger two, although they shared tasks rather evenly.

Health aides are not part of the cadre system; instead, they are health workers in a state-owned institution. These unskilled workers receive lower salaries than skilled or even semiskilled industrial workers. They begin at thirty-five yuan per month and only rarely make more. However, they receive free health care for themselves and their dependents and holiday, maternity, and retirement benefits. In addition, both younger health aides had recently been assigned their positions through *dingti*. The boy's mother had been a health aide on another ward in the hospital, and the girl's had been an aide in the hospital day-care center.

The training required for a health aide is minimal. The three aides on the infectious disease ward were lower or upper middle school graduates. Their tasks required some knowledge of sanitation and sterilization procedures but were otherwise janitorial. (See appendix 6 for details of their daily schedule.) During the Cultural Revolution, all nonphysician personnel were recruited as health aides and received on-the-job training that allowed them to move into other jobs. During that unstable period, people with little formal education but strong personal motivation were able to advance; a few even entered medical school. By 1980, however, the limitations of a weak basic foundation were recognized. Although an attempt was being made to help the health aides and former health aides to participate in the nursing or medical technician qualifying examination, most agreed that the rapid mobility of the past was over. One nurse claimed that "the health aid can still do anything. He can study hard and become a nurse or a technician; even a doctor." Yet several physicians were skeptical. "There is no foundation to build on," said one. "What point is there in their studying?" Despite this negative prediction, all three of the ward's health aides were taking part in the classes for promotion. At night the two younger aides met after supper on the ward and used the physicians' offices to study English and other subjects. If they do well, they may become nurses' aides, with fewer cleaning and more patient care duties. This advancement, of course, will depend on the work unit's need for a specific kind of worker.

Medical Technicians

The small laboratory located next to the infectious disease ward is a branch of the main hospital laboratory and conducts tests for the ward. During our stay the head of laboratories was assigned there, and two other technicians rotated through.[6]

6. It was hard to know whether this was a usual number of technicians or whether they were there because we were. Certainly the head of laboratories was initially assigned to the infectious disease lab because of our presence.

The head of laboratories, a man in his sixties, had been trained in laboratory research at a medical school but spent the twenty years following the 1957 Anti-Rightist Campaign sweeping hospital floors. Restored to his position at last, he was given pleasant housing in the hospital apartments and earned a salary of 100 yuan per month. His title was "teacher of technicians" (*jishi*). The other two technicians were a young man and a woman in her forties. The woman had been trained at a three-year vocational school following graduation from lower middle school in 1959. Until 1979 she had worked at Hubei's First Attached Hospital, and lived there with her husband, a physician. Her transfer was based on the Second Attached Hospital's need for more technicians, and she was being trained for a new kind of work that she felt would be interesting. It is apparently easier to negotiate transfers of personnel between hospitals attached to the same unit (in this case the medical college) than between unrelated units. Technicians (*jishi*) usually begin at forty yuan per month and can rise to eighty. She made about fifty yuan.

The young man was most commonly seen receiving instructions from the head of laboratories. He was a technical worker (*jishuyuan*) and had entered the job with no previous training. Technical workers initially earn thirty-six yuan per month and may receive over fifty yuan at the end of their careers, but this is rare. Not surprisingly, there is a backlog of medical technical workers waiting to be promoted to medical technicians, whose job they are actually performing. During the Cultural Revolution, technicians, like nurses, entered at this lower level and received on-the-job training. Technicians are all studying for the promotional examinations. The ladder is quite short, however. Beyond the level of medical technician, promotion is difficult.

In the medical school, one technician who had done cell biology and herpes virus research for twenty years had recently passed the examination to become a postgraduate student in the same laboratory. The other students accepted into this program were all medical school graduates. Such a promotion, however, is probably unusual. Several of the medical technicians seemed to feel their advancement potential was limited. One young woman who had been doing virology lab work for four years said, "Really the only way to be promoted is to be a technician teacher with responsibility for other technicians in the lab. But in the lab here, I am still under the control of the M.D., who wants to do research. I can't go higher without more training. I can't even really teach technicians because the teachers in those schools all have medical school degrees."

THE DAILY ROUTINE

At 8:00 A.M. promptly, five physicians and five of the eleven nurses assigned to the infectious disease ward assemble at the nursing station to hear morning report, given by the nurse and physician on duty the night before. The status of each patient is reviewed. A nurse is praised by the head nurse for her diligence in memorizing each patient's temperature for the morning recital. Special announcements concerning the ward or the hospital in general are made. Complaints or criticisms are heard. After about half an hour, each staff person moves to begin the morning's work, joining the three health aides, who have just returned from breakfast.

On this particular day, morning report is a busy half hour. One of the patients on the ward is a fifty-six-year-old man suffering from epidemic hemorrhagic fever. He has been very ill for about two weeks and is finally convalescing. The night nurse reports that during the night he pulled out his nasogastric tube and demanded food. Everyone laughs. Head Nurse Wang follows the night nurse's report with a summary of the annual meeting of the Chinese Academy of Nursing, which she recently attended in Beijing, and of new regulations for nurses. "Nurses should study English and other courses and take the examinations this spring. Our training during the Cultural Revolution was inadequate. We only know how to give shots and medicine, but we don't understand the principles behind our actions. I support this, but personally I don't want to study English—I'm too old." This brings a laugh from her staff. "It was also decided that in the future, each ward should have a nurse specially concerned with financial affairs. Also, patients and their relatives, especially their relatives, have criticized nurses, saying that they aren't taking good enough care of the patients." This information provokes heated discussion among both nurses and physicians. Several nurses argue that they cannot give better care unless more nurses are assigned to the ward; the ward should have fourteen nurses assigned, instead of eleven. Finally, the head nurse praises the behavior of a physician. "We all should look to Dr. Gao as a model. He volunteers for night duty before anyone has time to ask him. He never complains." As morning report ends, a physician from internal medicine enters with a brief announcement. It seems that the ward staff must choose doctors and nurses who have been good and bad examples and submit their names to the hospital as model workers, and workers who deserve criticism. They also should submit the names of those who were sick and off work a lot, and those who were not. When he finishes, morning report is over, and people break up into smaller groups to discuss issues raised or how the morning's work will proceed.

The physicians move to the ward rooms to begin morning rounds. Each doctor attends to his or her six to eight patients. All patients with the same disease are assigned to the same physician. Twice a week the head nurse accompanies the department chief on more formal rounds. On this particular day, we are asked to see several interesting cases, so we put on our white coats and hats and walk across the hall to the second patient ward room. Six or seven physicians and nurses, we two foreigners, and one medical college English teacher (equipped with a dictionary of medical terms) encircle the bed of a dysentery patient whose relatives have requested that he be examined by the American physician. The case is discussed openly in this setting; meanwhile several ambulatory patients rise from their beds to join the circle.

As the physicians move to the next patient ward room, the treatment shift nurses take over, taking temperatures, giving injections, updating medicine cards, and passing out the morning's medication from a dark wooden tray with forty holes for tiny porcelain pill cups. For each bed, a small order card is carefully filled out by the chief shift nurse, checked by another nurse, and taken to the pharmacy to be filled. When it is ready, the chief shift nurse picks it up and distributes the medicine according to the number on the tray next to the porcelain cup. Several nurses "make sure that each patient really swallows the medicine." (See duties of chief shift nurse, appendix 1). Those on the general nursing shift perform more mundane tasks such as changing the bedding, washing the seriously ill patients, sterilizing used equipment and laundry, and counting and checking a variety of items. Meanwhile the health aides circulate, taking lunch and dinner orders from all the patients, mopping the floors, and cleaning bathrooms.

In the next patient ward room an epidemic hemorrhagic fever patient is listed in critical condition. Because he is dehydrated, a nurse stands by his bed, pushing the IV fluid tubing with her fingers so that it will move faster. This patient was originally admitted to internal medicine for observation, with symptoms of headache, body ache, and vomiting blood. Several heads of internal medicine were unable to offer a diagnosis, so one of the infectious disease physicians was invited to consult. She immediately recognized the complex as epidemic hemorrhagic fever, but deferred diagnosis. She said, "When I saw that the internal medicine department heads hadn't been able to diagnose it, I went and got my department head to make the final diagnosis." This patient is semicomatose and has had hiccups for two days.

Unable to cure this symptom, the infectious disease physician asks for a consultation from the combined traditional and Western medicine ward. The chief shift nurse sends the order for a consultation, and soon thereafter a young M.D. appears on the ward with acupuncture needles to treat the man's hiccups. Meanwhile the physicians begin to disperse to the nursing station or to their office to write in the patient charts. As we leave the room, a nurse is attempting to give an injection to one of the patients. The patient asks if he must have it, because his neck is full of little bumps. The nurse hesitates and one of the physicians walks over and tells the patient that indeed he must accept the shot. The patient does not resist further. We back out of the door to the ward room, careful not to touch the door, and those who have had contact with patients in the room stop to soak their hands in the basin directly outside the ward.

After rounds, we gather in the physicians' office to discuss diagnoses and other aspects of patient care on the ward. As we talk, the interaction among the five physicians is lively and natural. Although the others defer to the chief of the section for final decisions on the ward, the conversations reflect an easy give-and-take that contradicts the authority relationship. Each seems to feel free to volunteer his or her opinions, perhaps in part because the chief has only recently been promoted to her position. She is only slightly older and more experienced than her colleagues. She is not a party member. She seems, in fact, to be a rather shy person who does not want to make radical changes in her new role. On the other hand, when the vice-director of the hospital in charge of medical treatment, and official head of infectious disease, enters the ward for his occasional rounds, the gentle camaraderie evaporates. He is older and more experienced than the other physicians on the ward, and he is a party member. His rank is several levels above that of most of the doctors. His presence has the effect of silencing the sardonic comments, joking, and mix of opinions that normally occur. He is the ultimate administrative authority over the functioning of the ward and its staff. This fact is reinforced by the constant repetition of "The director must decide." Because of his position as both hospital vice-director and infectious disease specialist, it is difficult to avoid deferring to his medical decisions. His low profile on the ward, however, kept this from becoming a viable issue for observation.

At eleven, the health aides stand outside the double doors at the end of the ward and call for the head nurse to come and unlock the doors. They wheel in the patients' food cart, and those who are able come to the door of their ward room with cup and bowl in hand to receive lunch. Patients too ill to get out of bed are served by the nurses and health aides. By quarter to twelve, all the ward staff except the few remaining on duty during noontime go home for lunch and a rest.

The ward is very quiet when we return from the noon meal. Most of the physicians have been called to meetings in their separate specialties to discuss hospitalwide examples of poor medical treatment. One such case involves a man who suffered acute renal failure as a result of an automobile accident and died as he was shuffled back and forth from radiology to the examination room in the outpatient department.

During the afternoon, we join the nurses as they perform their duties. Three nurses sit at the desks in the center of the nursing station. Two are making cotton swabs. From a large pile of cotton, one nurse pulls out identical swatches for the next nurse to wind around a small wooden stick with glue on the end. Hundreds are made in such a session. The third nurse is sitting beside a pile of metal chart cases, carefully recording daily temperatures. Noting that the physicians are off discussing the resolution of medical errors, we ask the nurses and the head nurse, who has just walked in, how such things are dealt with in the nursing profession. "For example," we say, "are nurses ever fired for poor performance? In the United States, a head nurse might dislike a certain nurse and simply fire her when she made a mistake." "Not here," replies the head nurse. "We will talk about it together. We help a nurse change, improve her abilities. If she makes a very serious mistake, perhaps she will take a rest for several months and resume her duties after that. If she is truly dangerous, I suppose the government would assign her to a different kind of job. But that is very rare."

It takes a special person to fulfill successfully the requirements of a job such as head nurse (see Fox and Swazey, forthcoming). As supervisor of both nurses and health aides, she must be a sympathetic friend, an enthusiastic supporter of what is often monotonous, menial work, *and* a stern public critic of any flaws she perceives in her staff or the functioning of the ward. She recognizes that much of the work is boring and that dissatisfaction is a natural response. But she feels that a positive attitude will counteract such feelings. "Sure, some people aren't happy—they want to give the orders instead of always being the ones to carry them out. But our work is work which must be done. We must have a good attitude about it. It is important." The formal methods of criticism at morning report appear to be an acceptable vehicle for correcting minor transgressions. She told us that serious problems are also discussed in the open, although probably following private discussions. "These must be aired," she said. "We are all working here together." Although we did not have the opportunity to observe this process, her approach to problems that arose on the ward concerning we Americans was straightforward. The resolution of serious problems in such a highly ritualized system may in fact depend much on personal style. The head nurse is a no-nonsense person who believes in speaking her mind, and the atmosphere on the ward is very informal. This informality extends to the health aides, who help the nurses with many of their tasks and participate in the give-and-take between them.

Xiao Shi is the baby of the ward. He is seventeen and all the nurses know that his mother, a recently retired hospital worker, is worried about his working on a ward that admits infectious disease patients. His father is a printer at the medical college, and they live in medical college housing. At three o'clock Xiao Shi and Xiao Li, the other young health aide, come back to work on the ward. They pour fresh water into the patients' thermoses, clean, dust, and help the nurses with their jobs. Xiao Shi offers to buy fruit or bread for patients who are walking about, saying that there are several vendors at the front of the hospital. The patients crowd to their ward room doors with money to give him. As the only male among so many women, he is teased and petted. It is unclear whether he will stay in this job for long or will move to another. He says he likes the work and is happy on the ward. At half past four, he and Xiao Li go to get the metal food cart at the patients' kitchen and bring it back to the ward. The head nurse unlocks the double doors, the patients are fed, and by half past five the health aides and the day-shift nurses are on their way home.

The few times we visited the ward at night, it seemed very quiet and dark. After supper, the patients are cared for by one nurse, with a physician on call. The ward television is rotated each evening, and patients read or knit. By nine the lights are out and the patients asleep. At half past one the evening-shift nurse is replaced by the night-shift nurse, who introduces the patients' conditions at morning report the next day.

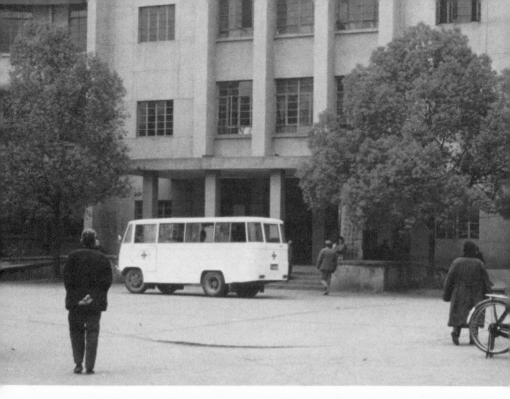

Main entrance of the Second Attached Hospital.

Corridor leading to the infectious disease ward.

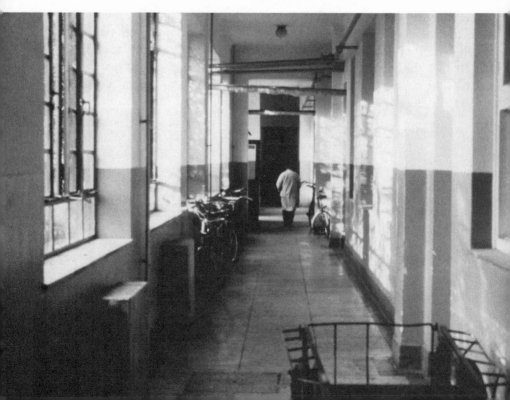

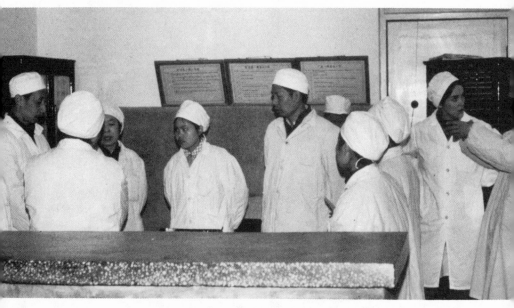

Morning report, which begins promptly at 8 A.M.

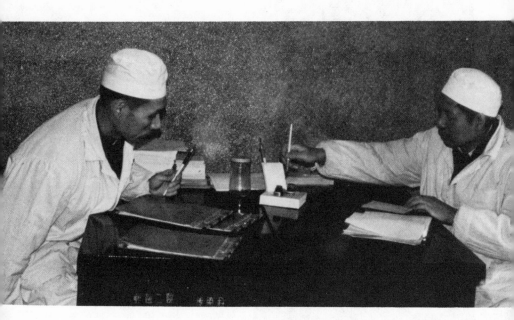

Physicians updating charts in their office.

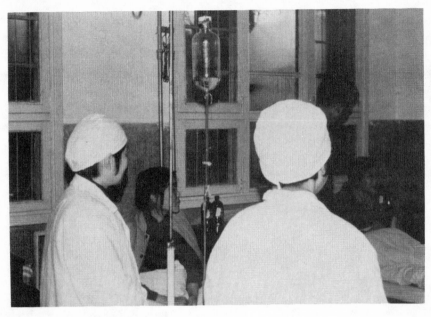

Ward rounds, generally held twice each week.

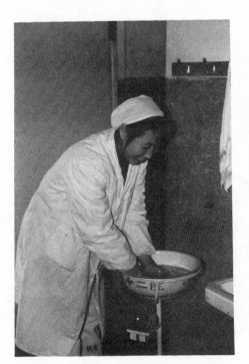

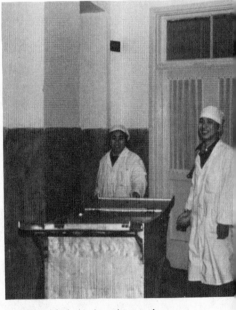

Health aids bringing the meal cart. Depending on the physicians' orders, patients are allowed to choose from two or three meals.

A nurse cleans her hands in a formaldehyde solution after examining a patient.

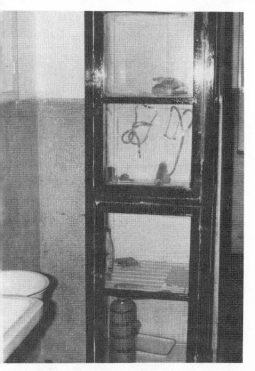

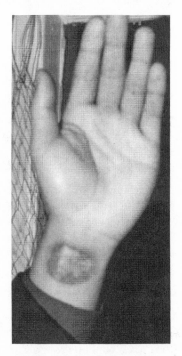

A hepatitis patient reveals the scar from moxibustion (cupping) performed by a neighbor to treat jaundice.

Shared stethoscopes are kept in a central cabinet where a basin of formaldehyde is allowed to evaporate.

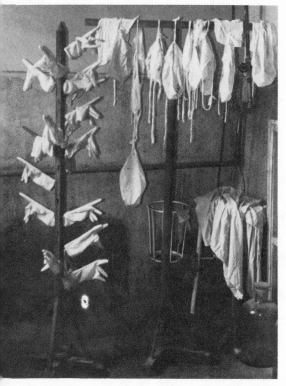

Gloves and masks are washed, dryed, and reused.

5

The Hospital, the Leaders, and the Professionals

THE HOSPITAL

The Second Attached Hospital (SAH) of Hubei Provincial Medical College (HPMC) contains the following departments: infectious disese, surgery, internal medicine, pediatrics, obstetrics and gynecology, neurology and urology, radiology, combined Western and traditional medicine, and ear, nose, throat, and dentistry. In addition, there is a special ward maintained for treatment of high-level cadres. Behind the hospital are facilities for cancer patients: a cancer inpatient building, a radiation therapy department, a nuclear medicine building, and a radiation therapy outpatient building that provides inexpensive patient facilities.[1] The SAH has 580 beds and 830 staff, including 300 physicians, 300 nurses, and 230 administrators, technicians, and workers. Salaries range from 35 to 200 yuan per month (only three staff are paid as much as 200 yuan); the average salary is approximately 63 yuan (U.S. $42).

The SAH admits 7,000 patients yearly. The average number of outpatients seen yearly is 370,000, or about 1,000 patients a day. The average stay for inpatients is nineteen days.[2] The First Attached Hospital of HPMC is slightly larger. Each year it admits almost 10,000 inpatients, with an average stay of slightly over nineteen days, and sees 575,000 outpatients (1,500 each day). The third facility attached to HPMC is a dental hospital that admits 1,000 inpatients and sees 128,000 outpatients yearly.

1. Called the "simple ward" (*jianyi bingfang*), it charges only .2 yuan per day for a room, in contrast to the hospital inpatient room fee of .7 yuan per day.
2. This is a longer average length of stay than that in other countries. The average in the United States is about nine days; in European countries it is somewhat higher (U.S. Department of Health, Education and Welfare 1976).

A comparable hospital in the United States, North Carolina Memorial Hospital (NCMH), in Chapel Hill, North Carolina, is a teaching hospital attached to the University of North Carolina School of Medicine.[3] It has 572 beds and 3,475 staff, including nurses, administrators, other personnel, and medical residents. Not included in this figure are 510 attending physicians whose salaries are paid through the medical college by funds generated from patient care and paid directly to the medical college. The average number of outpatients seen yearly at NCMH is 283,000, (755 per day). NCMH admits 20,000 patients yearly (55 patients per day), and the average stay for inpatients is 8.9 days. These figures, in combination with information presented in chapters 6 and 7, show clearly that hospitals of comparable size in the United States move patients through far more quickly. They accomplish this by employing larger staffs, marshaling a broader spectrum of technical diagnostic and curative tools, and relying more on convalescence at home.

ADMINISTRATION

In the words of one hospital administrator, the SAH is "directly led" by the medical college, which is in turn under the authority of the provincial bureaus of health and education (see figure 7). The hospital and medical college maintain separate administrations, and both are dependent upon provincial bureaus for major financial decisions, including budgets and staff salaries. Day-to-day affairs in the hospital are conducted independently, but any important policy or administrative decisions are under the control of the medical college leadership.

The hospital administration is headed by the director (*zheng yuanzhang*). At the SAH, he is a Communist party member and a physician. In addition to administration, he oversees medical education on the wards. Four vice-directors (*fuyuanzhang*) head the departments that conduct the business of running a hospital: Medical Treatment, led by a party member and physician trained in infectious disease; Medical Education, led by a party member and army veteran of Yanan;[4] and Administration and Gen-

3. Data on NCMH were obtained from interviews with Bill J. Fuller, Associate Director of Fiscal Services, North Carolina Memorial Hospital, 4 November 1981.

4. Yanan was Mao Zedong's guerrilla stronghold in northern China, from which he launched successful attacks against the Japanese and later the Nationalist army. Those who became involved with the Chinese Communist party movement during the Yanan days have greater status today. In the health field, we noted some correlation between experience in Yanan and appointment to a high-level administration post.

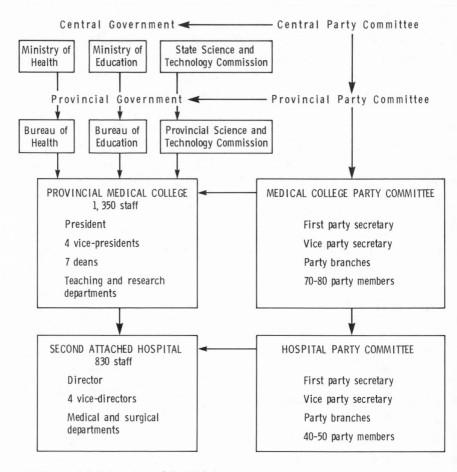

Figure 7. Administration of the Unit

eral Affairs, both headed by the same vice-director, whose background was unknown to us. A variety of assistants and subordinate offices carry out each department's functions.

The administration of the medical college corresponds to that of the hospital. The president of the college (*yuanzhang*) is a party member, a physician trained in pediatrics, and a veteran nurse of Yanan. Under her leadership, four vice-presidents oversee the medical college and the three attached hospitals: Personnel and the President's Office are headed by a party member whose educational background was unknown to us, Medical Education by a party member educated in law at the Chinese People's University, and Administration by a party member and veteran of the 1949 revolution. The fourth vice-president, a physician trained in obstetrics and gynecology, is not a party member. He is in charge of the medical college library and medical treatment in the three hospitals. Under these four departments are seven deans, two in the President's Office, three in the Medical Education Office (two in charge of medical education and one in charge of scientific research), and two in the Administration Department. The teaching departments (basic sciences, pediatrics, and medicine) are under the administration of the Medical Education Office.

Ultimately, the Chinese Communist party and its basic-level organizations at the hospital and medical college direct the implementation of all political and economic policies and address local concerns ranging from personnel appointments to teaching and research. Criteria for party membership have varied over time. During the Cultural Revolution, political attitude was paramount. Today, hard work and achievement on the job seem most important. While we were in China, application to the party was being promoted for the many middle-aged intellectuals who did not have the opportunity to join during the Cultural Revolution.[5]

The party organizations in the hospital and medical college are separate, although the medical college party leaders have authority over those of the hospital. In the SAH, forty to fifty party members are dispersed among the various departments and service organs and grouped into several party branch organizations. The party committee of the hospital is headed by the first party secretary, who is also the director of the hospital. The vice–party secretary post is filled by one of the hospital vice-directors. The medical college, with 1,350 staff, has more party members, perhaps seventy to eighty, composing several party branches.[6] The positions of first and vice–party secretaries of the medical college party committee are also filled by the college president and one of the vice-presidents, respectively.[7]

5. We were told that applications were turned in by most of the teachers in basic sciences, for example. These applications were then processed by party members in the individual's small group (*xiaozu*) at work. The applicant would be interviewed and observed, with evaluation based on criteria such as competence, punctuality, and effort. Political criteria were not mentioned. Those not admitted to the party were informed of the reasons by a party leader and their applications kept on file for future consideration.

6. In the English department, for example, there are three party members. Their branch organization is composed of party members from the English, physics, and chemistry departments and is subordinate to the medical college party committee.

7. Before the Cultural Revolution, the first party secretary and the president of the college were often the same person, especially if the president was also a party member, although at that time it was not essential for the president to belong to the party. Likewise, during the Cultural Revolution, the president was both vice–party secretary and vice-president of the col-

This telescoping of administrative and political leadership roles is a common though unintentional characteristic of the *danwei* system.[8] The effect at the local level is to place a great deal of power in the hands of a few unit and party leaders. Furthermore, when the party administrator is a nonprofessional, concentration of power may create conflicts for nonparty professionals working in the organization. In the medical college, for example, more than half of the top posts were occupied by nonprofessional party members. In the hospital, however, and in the medical college departments directly concerned with medicine, the administrative posts were more commonly filled by party physicians. In the aftermath of the Cultural Revolution, professionals have been encouraged to take on administrative responsibility. The central government has addressed the problem of overconcentration of administrative power in party hands by recommending that administrative and party posts be filled separately (Pepper 1981). Despite these policy changes, the majority of newly promoted administrators in the hospital and medical college units seem to combine professional qualifications and party membership.

FINANCE

The hospital Finance Department has authority to make decisions about very few important matters. Rather, the SAH appears to function as a financial conduit between the state and the clients it serves.

First, as mentioned earlier, the hiring of staff and consequent changes in budget allocation for staff salaries are controlled by the provincial government. All staff salaries in the hospital are provided for in the provincial budget, and the provincial bureau allocates all medical personnel in accordance with its perception of the staff requirements of all hospitals under its jurisdiction. The hospital may apply each year for new staff assignments, but the final decision rests with the state.

---

lege. The president and the first party secretary were attacked and overthrown by the Red Guards for "protecting intellectuals." The first party secretary was later given a job in the provincial government, and the president promoted to her current job, while another was named first party secretary. The latter also returned to provincial government work, so during our stay the president was filling both posts on a provisional basis. Soon after we left, there was to be a meeting of the medical college party members to elect the committee. The president would probably be elected to her current position of first party secretary.

8. Franz Schurmann (1966, 156) has noted that "by 1958, most positions of organizational leadership were held by Party members. They, therefore, functioned in a dual capacity: they were cadres in some working unit and they were also Party cadres. Nevertheless, the Chinese Communists have never formally merged the two roles."

Second, the hospital budget and economic plan for each year are also established by the provincial government, based on assessment of previous performance. The SAH revenue from patient fees for 1979 was 1,920,000 yuan (U.S. $1,267,200). This sum accounted for approximately 63 percent of the total cost of running the hospital, including medicines (900,000 yuan, or 47 percent of patient bills), small equipment (180,000 yuan, or 9 percent of patient bills), room, heat, laboratory, radiology, supplies, and small overhead costs. These items are charged to patients on their hospital bills and are paid directly to the provincial government. The remaining hospital costs, calculated at approximately 1,130,000 yuan (U.S. $753,000), or 37 percent of the total budget, are provided for elsewhere in the provincial government budget. The provincial contribution covers staff salaries (630,000 yuan), large-equipment costs of over 10,000 yuan, administrative costs (4 yuan per month per physician assigned, or about 14,400 yuan), building repair (2 yuan per square meter of building), deficit spending (200 yuan per bed, or 116,000 yuan), and a sum to assist patients who are unable to pay their hospital bills (50 yuan per bed per year).[9] Together, the revenue derived directly from patient care charges (1,920,000 yuan) and the sums allocated in the provincial budget (1,130,000 yuan) result in a total annual operating budget of approximately 3,050,000 yuan (U.S. $2,013,000).

Although private hospitals in the United States have much more budgetary flexibility, the state-run North Carolina Memorial Hospital is remarkably similar to the SAH. Close state regulation of the NCMH budget, with its line-item budget,[10] limits the financial decisions of hospital administrators. In fact, one administrator indicated that his role resembled that of a financial middleman, similar to that of the SAH administrators. The NCMH total budget is $98,200,000 (or about fifty times the size of the SAH budget). Over half (59 percent) of this budget goes to staff salaries and benefits, compared with one-fourth of the SAH budget. Patient receipts, which are paid monthly to the state government, cover 72.2 percent of all expenses, and 20 percent of the budget is subsidized by the state legislature.[11]

9. The estimate of the total provincial contribution reported to us during our stay was as follows: 630,000 yuan for staff salaries, and a maximum additional allocation of 500,000 yuan to supplement patient fees.

10. Line-item budgeting does not allow money to be transferred from one item (such as supplies or salaries) to another. Money can, however, be transferred within categories.

11. This large subsidy is necessary primarily because NCMH, as a state hospital, is obliged to admit all patients, particularly indigents, whom private hospitals will not accept. Most hospitals in the United States must meet their budgets through patient fees.

Clearly, government-controlled hospitals are not profit-generating institutions. When questioned about the difficulty of meeting such a tightly structured budget, the SAH administrators cited several additional sources of income that are available directly to the hospital and that seem to be used at the local level. One is registration fees for outpatient and inpatient care (.05 yuan per visit, totaling 18,600 yuan per year at the SAH). A second source of discretionary funds is profit from the sale of medicines—50 percent on Western medicines, and 20–30 percent on traditional herbs.[12] The hospital currently buys most of its drugs from the government, but when the construction of its pharmaceutical factory is complete, it will produce its own medicines for less and thus increase its profit. Third, because the SAH is a teaching hospital, all investments made for purposes of medical education are paid for by the medical college. The newly constructed nuclear medicine building, for example, was built by the college because its purpose is teaching and research. Although it was impossible to estimate the amount of these discretionary funds, they undoubtedly represent a small proportion of the entire budget.

The medical college also is heavily dependent on the provincial bureaus for finance and management decisions, including staff salaries and assignments. Tuition fees, admission criteria, student curriculum, and other recent changes in medical education are all national or provincial policy decisions. In research there is some individual decision making, but the major input is from the national and provincial government.[13] Most areas of medical research are established by the Ministry of Health, in Beijing. HPMC, for example, was named by the ministry as one of the major centers for the study of epidemic hemorrhagic fever and the relationship between herpes virus and cervical cancer. Other research topics are named by the provincial bureaus, and a few are decided by individual teachers or researchers. Funding for these projects comes through the Ministry of Health and three sources in the provincial government: the Bureau of Education, the Bureau of Health, and the Science and Technology Commission. Each year, funding proposals are made by the medical college departments or research institutes, submitted to the medical college for approval, and reviewed by pro-

12. Some money from sales of medicine is used to offset the cost of care in other areas, such as operating-room costs. A chest operation, for example, costs ninety yuan, but patients are charged only fifty.

13. Another demonstration of the state's control over research decisions occurred when we contacted leaders at Wuhan Medical College, a nationally run school, to discuss research topics for exchanges between it and Yale. We were told that the topics would be selected only by the Ministry of Health, not by local researchers.

vincial-level committees. Long-term projects are reviewed and funded in accordance with the recommendations of these groups. Some of the provincial officials are scientists themselves, but many are not. When asked about the problems involved when scientific projects are evaluated by non-scientists, one of the college researchers said, "Some of the nonscientists can see farther than others. Many know science is important. They receive our suggestions and they listen. But we don't complain about their decisions." Nevertheless, he described an incident four years earlier, when funds for a long-term research project under his direction had been threatened. His research team argued with the Science and Technology Commission about the need to continue the work, and the funds were spared.[14] In addition, the researcher noted that the medical college has a special science commission, composed of four to ten scientists, organized to discuss scientific work and to communicate their ideas to the leaders of the medical college. The bargaining power of scientists in such funding decisions has risen dramatically since the anti-intellectual Cultural Revolution.

THE LEADERS

In chapter 3 we examined the role of the leaders in the daily life of *danwei* members. Here we examine the relationship between leaders and staff members at work.

References to the administrative and work group leadership as "the leaders" or "our leaders" (*women de lingdaoren*) are ubiquitous, as though the leaders were one undifferentiated mass.[15] Although individual staff members tend to identify with the leader or leaders directly responsible for their work, there is a definite perception of the leadership as a composite

14. In a paper discussing research and development in industrial enterprises in China, William A. Fischer argues that the lack of technical training of administrative cadres who are responsible for funding research projects has had the effect of reducing their ability to control those funds: "One . . . frequently finds that *all projects submitted from below to an R&D administrative organ are automatically approved* (Fischer 1981, 19; emphasis added).

Although Fischer does not comment on how much independence there is in the initiation of research proposals (and we suspect there are many that are assigned by authorities from above), his observations confirm that local-level scientists have some influence on decisions.

15. China now suffers from an overabundance of leaders in many spheres. After the Cultural Revolution, many old cadres were rehabilitated and only the top leaders from the preceding decade were removed from their positions. That policy left many middle- and lower-level administrators trying to fill too few jobs. Several of our unit members laughingly repeated to us a common description of how things had changed at HPMC: "Before the Cultural Revolution all the leaders could fit into one classroom. Now they could not fit into two." In an attempt to solve this problem, retirement is being recommended for many of the older cadres.

whole, responsible *together* for governing the unit. One member of the *danwei* defined collective leadership in the following way: "Collective leadership means that it's not just one person running things. And, moreover, when a person is a leader he does not represent himself, but represents the organization. We Chinese say, 'Rely upon the organization and believe in the masses' (*yikao zuzhi, xiangxin chunzhong*)." Ideally, a leader does not pursue self-aggrandizement but acts as a representative of the organization. Problems were said to occur when the leader tries to create an "independent kingdom" or, conversely, when collective leadership comes to mean collective shirking of individual responsibility for decisions or policy implementation.

Work units are hierarchical, bureaucratic organizations whose staff are assigned and whose leaders are appointed.[16] Some institutionalized mechanisms for democratic feedback from the *danwei* members to their leaders have been developed. The one most commonly cited is "consultation with the masses" whenever major plans or policies are being considered. These consultations may take place in small work groups such as the infectious disease ward staff. For example, at one morning report the new economic campaign was explained to the staff and their opinions solicited. Strong feelings about the proposed staff-to-bed ratio were freely offered, and the staff planned to request another physician and nurse for the ward. To our knowledge, the ratio was not changed. At another morning report, criticisms of patient care were relayed and the staff were given a chance to respond. For decisions on the ward itself, staff members are generally given a chance to participate in discussions about an upcoming change. In addition to group discussions, special days for criticism are regularly scheduled. Every year at Spring Festival, the leaders of the hospital circulate to hear criticisms of their performance. Likewise, monthly meetings are scheduled between patients and staff to hear patient complaints. Finally, although we did not have access to these meetings, the political small-group discussions held among the ward staff every Tuesday afternoon were used for debate of local issues in addition to the usual discussion of political campaigns, *People's Daily* articles, and other national issues.

Consultations also occur between higher levels; in fact these are considered to be the backbone of the centralized system of economic planning in

16. While we were in China, experiments with the democratic election of cadres were just beginning. People in our unit had heard of such events, but they were not directly involved. If elections are in fact widely implemented, they will offer another significant institutionalized mechanism for bottom-up influence in units.

China. Thus, the budgets of the hospital and the medical college are not merely imposed by the provincial bureaus. Rather, central planners propose a budget and send it to local-level units for their input. There are limits to the power of work unit leaders to influence changes in the proposed budgets. Campaigns to alter financial allocations such as we witnessed at our hospital are further evidence of the control that the state exercises over the local level. Still, as we saw in the funding of medical research projects, lower levels do alter central decisions, and campaigns can be successful only with the cooperation of the units.

The formal participation of *danwei* members in work-related decisions contradicts the picture of authoritarian unit leadership and centralized control of units from above. Yet it is difficult to evaluate the significance of these mechanisms for the people involved. Presumably, participation increases an individual's sense of efficacy and loyalty to the organization. As short-term members of the *danwei*, we were impressed by the belief expressed by *danwei* friends that their input made a genuine difference in unit affairs. Yet Etzioni (1975, 167–68) has pointed out that such mechanisms may also conceal manipulation, acting to co-opt people into loyalty to the organization by giving them a sense of participation. Hirschman (1970) also noted this mode of extracting loyalty, which then influences the individual's choice of exit or voice.

If unit leaders ignore feedback from lower levels, other options are available for expressing grievances. Hirschman proposed that, in general, dissatisfied organizational members have two choices, to leave (exit) and to complain (voice). In his view, when exit is difficult or impossible, complaints become more frequent. In examining a nonmarket (no-exit) situation, the Polish economy, Kolarska and Aldrich (1980) reach the opposite conclusion.[17] They agree that those who are not free to leave necessarily have a greater investment in the organization and that formal mechanisms established to communicate complaints do encourage their expression. Nevertheless, they assert that when members are unable to leave an organization, the use of voice leaves them vulnerable to retaliation from the leadership. Furthermore, in a nonmarket setting, although voice may grow, its *impact* may be blunted by the increased power of the organization over its members (Kolarska and Aldrich 1980). In other words, because the members are forced to remain in the organization, the leaders may not need to be as responsive to complaints as they might be if the members could threaten them

17. Kolarska and Aldrich base some of their arguments on Barry (1974), Birch (1975), and Laver (1976).

with exit. Kolarska and Aldrich also introduce the notion (which we will discuss below) that if direct appeals to organizational leaders are less effective under no-exit conditions, members may turn more frequently to authorities outside the organization.

We lived and worked in our unit for several months before we began to understand the dynamics of conflict resolution and decision making. In our roles as teachers and members of the infectious disease ward staff, we were allowed to participate in a variety of official discussions and informal meetings. At the formal meetings, convened for the specific purpose of making decisions about some issue, no one but the leaders talked. A predictable agenda emerged. Everyone sat down; the leader, in the center, announced the topic and asked for opinions; none were offered and the leader announced the decision. In our classes and on the ward, when we attempted to generate discussion about decisions that had to be made, the response often consisted of silence or a shifting about in chairs, and eventually someone rose to say that they would discuss it later. We were confused. Were the leaders really as unilateral and the staff members as uncomfortable with group discussion as they seemed?

Gradually it dawned upon us that all the discussions had taken place behind the scenes, and that the formal meetings we witnessed were simply the conclusions of earlier debates. As one American researcher recently engaged in the training of enterprise managers in China put it, "Before scheduled meetings to discuss our progress, the managers would arrive and say, 'We've met. These are our recommendations.'"[18] In our own classes, we were demanding open discussions without allowing the students their own internal meetings. In doing so, we were asking them to circumvent a basic protective device. This device, whereby a particular group meets to decide upon a course of action, a recommendation, or a collective complaint, is the unit staff members' corollary to collective leadership. It is a kind of group voice that allows them to avoid individual responsibility for any opinion or decision. Under this protection, however, a delegate of such a group will not hesitate to express even the most embarrassing complaint.[19] More than once while walking in the *danwei* we suddenly met a staff member who casually said, "Our teaching group has had a meeting and appointed me as their spokesman. . . ." A complaint inevitably followed, and because it was

18. William A. Fischer, personal communication.
19. Feedback through a group representative is institutionalized throughout the educational system. Each class in the medical school chooses a monitor (*banzhang*) to act as its delegate and to represent its opinions or grievances.

the opinion of a group rather than of just one individual, it carried more weight.

Kolarska and Aldrich conclude that the use of indirect voice to contact an outside authority becomes increasingly common when exit is not an alternative. In our unit, we observed a ritualization of this process, through the formal procedure of "raising an opinion" (*tiyi*) to express grievances to a higher authority.[20] When staff members are frustrated in their dealings with lower-level leaders, they commonly turn to other leaders. On several occasions we asked staff members how an individual would lodge a complaint with the leadership. We received the following replies: "We go to the leader in question. If that doesn't work, then we might go to another leader and raise an opinion"; "If we can't get satisfaction, we might go to yet another leader, or even to the president of the medical college, face to face. She will listen if we want to talk to her"; "If some leader is trying to create an independent kingdom, then the people will of course criticize him or her to higher levels"; "Higher levels often investigate lower levels, too, to make sure they pay attention to the masses";[21] "We can write to the national leaders."[22]

When a problem arises for an individual unit member, it is also possible to contact leaders informally, to gain advice and help in working out a solution. For example, a young English teacher in the medical college applied to the college to be a candidate for a national examination to study medical English at another institution. He was told to wait for a year so that another member of the English department might have the opportunity to take the examination. He immediately sought out a third English teacher who had also been denied a chance the previous year but had somehow managed to take the examination anyway. He hoped that her strategy of appealing to another leader (actually several different leaders) would also be useful in reversing the decision on his own case.

Whether staff communicate directly or indirectly, they are dependent on the goodwill of their leaders for the effective functioning of feedback devices. Consequently they are vulnerable to abuses by leaders who are not re-

20. The use of indirect voice in appeals to outside authorities not in direct control over the leaders was mentioned occasionally, but it is rare today. Strategies such as writing letters to newspapers and appealing to the general public by posting the now-outlawed "big character posters" (*dazibao*), were the norm during the Cultural Revolution.

21. These investigations are formal events conducted by higher levels when a complaint is judged to be serious enough.

22. The last time any one we asked remembered writing to a national leader was in 1953. She did receive a reply.

sponsive to their appeals. Ironically, the reliance on goodwill rather than on institutionalized controls of local leaders parallels the Confucian scholar official (*zhunzi*) ideal.

Leaders have developed their own set of devices to deal with pressures from their staff. First, as mentioned earlier, leaders make decisions together. Although the ultimate authority for unit affairs rests with the party and the first party secretary,[23] collective leadership tends to prevent any one leader from assuming responsibility for any one decision. Second, leaders are removed from the initial arena of confrontation because those who implement decisions are rarely the ones who make them. The person responsible for conveying news of a decision by the leaders is usually a secretary or aide who can only take out a pocket notebook and carefully write down the complaints of those receiving the news. This procedure acts as an effective buffer, for a unit member is never quite sure how or when these notebooks are read.

Third, the most common response to complaints or requests from below seems to be no response. We observed several instances in which staff requests were answered by statements such as "We will look into the matter" but no further action was taken. Because the leaders had indicated that something would be done, it was difficult for the staff members to make further inquiries.

Finally, lower-level leaders do not view complaints to higher levels as negative. Rather, the existence of these channels allows them to pass along responsibility to someone with higher authority (and perhaps more funds or political security).

A PERSONAL ANECDOTE

Our work on the infectious disease ward and assignment to hospital staff housing meant that we were members (however temporary) of the hospital *danwei*, and under the authority of its leadership. We had close day-to-day contact with one hospital leader or with his administrative secretary. This leader had had no experience with foreign visitors and certainly did not know how we expected to be led. Likewise, our introduction to the unit was sudden and filled with new and unusual experiences. Although our lives could not be described as typical of our Chinese colleagues, the strategies

23. Again, there are plans to divest party administrators of some of their power. (Pepper 1981).

that we and the leader employed in our interactions illustrate several important points.

One of our chief aims was to conduct research on epidemic hemorrhagic fever, a disease that commonly required admission to our ward and that would be of interest to our American sponsors. To collect background information and review hospital records related to epidemic hemorrhagic fever, we requested the assistance of hospital physicians and of English teachers who might help with translation. We were operating from what seemed to be a position of strength: the medical college leaders seemed genuinely concerned that our visit be a success; we were trying to facilitate an exchange program that might prove of great benefit to the unit; we were also teaching English, which constituted a valuable service apart from our medical research goals. Somewhat naively, we foresaw no obstacles to our requests. We had regular meetings with the leader's secretary, who carefully recorded our progress and requests and promised rapid responses. After six weeks (and visits to every possible tourist attraction) we realized that (1) any work we performed had political and/or personal significance for our colleagues and the responsible leader, (2) any work our colleagues performed to assist us would require the leader's explicit consent, and (3) decisions regarding our work would be made by several leaders in collaboration.

At the same time, another incident occurred that spurred us to act. We had carefully trained our English teacher-translator to help us in our epidemic hemorrhagic fever project. This training involved expansion of her vocabulary and familiarity with chart reviews. However, her leader was interested in exposing all the English teachers to our accent, and so one morning in December a new translator appeared in her place; our first translator, who had predicted our infuriated response, made herself scarce. The hospital leader had no jurisdiction over the medical college English department. That morning we stormed into the office of a medical college leader whom we had met several times, a physician who acted as an assistant to the president of the medical college. We unloaded all our complaints and requests and insisted that he become our new leader. Our situation was an uncomfortable one: we knew that our aggression was unusual and feared it would offend our hosts; we also felt fondness and respect for our hospital leader, and we did not want to damage his position.

Our behavior had a variety of effects. First, our translator returned. Second, we and several physicians were allowed to begin work on epidemic hemorrhagic fever. Third, we amused our Chinese colleagues by our attempt to identify a leader of our choice. Fourth, we learned a critical lesson:

it was permissible to go around a leader. His powers were limited, and he was probably relieved rather than harmed by diffusion of responsibility for decisions. Finally, our Chinese colleagues seemed impressed by our commitment, and from our perspective (and as far as we know) the whole episode ended in a positive light.

WORK AUTONOMY ON THE WARD

Work autonomy is the freedom to determine what knowledge will be used in one's job and how that knowledge will be applied (Montagna 1977, 167). Some occupations are inherently more autonomous than others. Physicians have more input into the nature of their jobs than do nurses, who typically allow others to define the knowledge they apply. In China, considering the degree of administrative control over both the work unit system and the system of health care delivery, one would predict a decrease in autonomy for hospital staff. Furthermore, in accordance with the government's egalitarian goals, the autonomy of the professional is subject to ideological as well as bureaucratic constraints.

The work autonomy of nurses on our ward was similar to that of nurses in the United States (Montagna 1977), except in two seemingly contradictory respects: nurses in China are more closely supervised, yet there is a stronger attempt to involve nurses in group decision making.

The allotted tasks of both nurses and health aides are clearly spelled out (see appendixes 1–3). Slogans on the wall enjoin staff to "Establish the Four Attitudes and the Four Strictnesses of Medical Work Style" (see appendix 4), and for the personnel on duty there are the "Five Not Allowed": "not allowed to come late or leave early, no absences without permission, not allowed to leave while on duty, not allowed to conduct private affairs while on duty, and don't put off today's work until tomorrow." Such rules are typical of all work organizations in China and are promulgated at the national level as well.[24] This predilection for establishing a set of rules to manage any task or situation recalls traditional Chinese codes of morality. Today in China, the correct performance of one's work is defined in socialist terms as a moral accomplishment. In the hospital, rules for nurses and other hospital staff are further elevated into a code of "medical morality" in which "traditional Chinese concepts and ethical principles, contemporaneous Chinese Socialist doctrine, and modern scientific and technological

24. See *Beijing Review* 25, no. 25 (28 July 1982):3 for an example of "rules for peasants."

premises are brought together" (Fox and Swazey, forthcoming; see also Garfield 1978).

Nurses thus perform their tasks in a rather rigid setting with an abundance of rules and closely conducted restraints on behavior and attitudes. Nevertheless, our own observations and those of others (Garfield 1978) indicate that relationships between nurses and physicians are friendly and more egalitarian than in Western hospitals. Doctors and nurses met together to discuss overnight patient problems, and nurses' opinions were carefully solicited. All the staff seemed to participate in discussions of policies and in at least some decisions that affected their jobs on the ward. Although some social distance was evident when high-level party officials came onto the ward, the general atmosphere was that of a team approach.

These egalitarian rituals do not offset physician control. In a recent analysis of a U.S.-Chinese nursing exchange program, Dirschel observed that

> nurses in China have little or no autonomy and little opportunity for decision making in patient care. The physician dominates. When the patient arrives at the hospital, the physician determines his degree of illness as well as his diagnosis. If he is very ill, he is assigned to a nurse who has a small caseload. The physician makes all the decisions; nurses provide the care. (1981)

Nursing in China is characterized by both traditional and socialist elements not found in the United States. As in the American system, rewards in the organization involve increased responsibility for administrative tasks rather than increased autonomy in the area of medical care; although nurses are treated with respect, they are never recognized as professional equals (Bates 1978). These appear to be features of the occupation, independent of the health care system or the *danwei*. Our observations and those of others (Fox and Swazey, forthcoming), however, indicate that nursing may be a profession in transition; nurses may achieve more autonomy if they are able to define work that they alone are qualified to perform.

In the case of physicians, it is easier. In order to disentangle the determinants of occupation from the influence of the health care and the unit systems. Because physicians typically enjoy the greatest work autonomy of any occupation, their conflicts with the hospital bureaucracy (the organization's tendency to rationalize and supervise knowledge and tasks) and the hospital leaders should reveal more about the extent of control over work in the *danwei*.

Studies of hospital organizations in the United States have shown that the presence of physicians introduces important changes in the basic functioning of an organization. Smith (1955) defined the problem as a built-in conflict springing from a dual authority system invested in lay administrators and professionals who often have different objectives. Goss (1963) argued that the incorporation of professionals and their values actually changes the nature of authority relations in an organization. She proposed that in the realm of administrative work, formal authority relations persisted, whereas in professional work hierarchical relations were advisory; hence the hospital organization is an "advisory bureaucracy."[25] Freidson (1970a) demonstrated that physicians in hospital organizations in the United States maintain considerable autonomy vis-à-vis the supervision of administrators, who tend to treat doctors in a conciliatory manner. Given that physicians attached to hospital organizations in the United States have many exit options, in addition to the strength they derive from their technical competence, this degree of autonomy is hardly surprising.

With few exceptions, private practice in China is not allowed, and doctors are assigned to work under the direct control and supervision of hospital administrators. In contrast, in a country like the United States, private practice (with practically no supervision) is the norm, and even physicians employed in hospital organizations may be members of protective guildlike associations, such as the American Medical Association, which exist outside of and often in opposition to the hospital organization (Johnson 1972).

In terms of employment alternatives within the national bureaucratic organization, physicians in China are in a poor position: their salary, benefits, housing, and potential to generate additional income are all set by the state. Funding for medical research projects is approved through the same channels, although usually the medical college teachers and researchers play a role in application for research funds. Physicians, even in a teaching hospital such as the SAH, are limited to the practice of medicine.

Another factor influencing the autonomy of physicians is the power derived from membership in the Chinese Communist party. In the Soviet Union, Field found that party membership "transcends all other considerations and contributes to undermining cooperation among medical personnel and to upset lines of authority" (1957, 125; see also Knaus 1981). He ob-

25. Goss defines *advisory* as "the right to give advice that subordinates are obliged to take under consideration but not necessarily to follow in making their decisions" (1953, 177). These two relationships are distinguished in Chinese as an "authority relationship" (*lingdao guanxi*) and "advisory relationship" (*zhuanye guanxi*).

served that nonparty Soviet physicians deferred to party physicians in medical and other matters. Furthermore, the common practice of placing nonphysician party members in administrative posts over nonparty physicians (when not enough party physicians were available) further contributed to the difficulties between professionals and administrators.

The role of the party in our unit was similar. Many administrators in the hospital and medical college are party members. A few are also nonprofessionals, although the trend seems to be toward appointing administrators who are both party members and physicians. Our limited observations of the interaction between physicians and administrators provide several tentative conclusions. First, party membership is a definite advantage for professional career advancement. We were told on several occasions that party membership increases the power of a physician or scientist, particularly when discretionary funding decisions are involved.[26] Likewise, a physician or scientist who is not a party member may be handicapped, especially in appointments to leadership positions.[27] Finally, although we had no opportunity to observe physicians interacting with nonprofessional administrators, we did observe that nonparty physicians generally defer to party physicians in positions of authority. Party membership thus provides administrators with an extra source of control over professionals within the unit.

Despite constraints on the power of physicians in China, their position within the medical care system was sufficiently strong to provoke prolonged criticism during the Cultural Revolution. Physicians were attacked for authoritarian relationships with patients and with medical staff. There was a nationally publicized attempt to redistribute power in the medical system through "sharing" the information and skills that physicians generally control. During this time, visitors to China enthusiastically reported that China had "deprofessionalized" the role of the physician (Sidel and Sidel 1973).[28]

Descriptions of the practice of medicine during the Cultural Revolu-

26. For example, if a physician applies to the hospital for a new piece of equipment, party membership increases the chances of approval.

27. Two cases illustrate these points. In one, the cochair of a medical school department was a forty-year-old party member who had risen to her position during the Cultural Revolution. Her former teacher, a sixty-year-old noted scientist, had only recently been named cochair with her and was resentful of the power that the younger woman still had over him. The second case involved the department of internal medicine in the hospital. The department head, a party member and physician, was named over eight other vice-chairs, many of whom were technically more qualified but few of whom were party members.

28. The motivation behind these changes in nursing tasks corresponds to efforts in the United States to "professionalize" nursing. The difference is that in China the goal was to

tion indicate that rather than a genuine elimination of physician dominance, there were sporadic attacks upon their power accompanied by a general breakdown in the supervision of medical practice. Thus, in the hospitals, most physicians swept floors but also continued to take care of patients. Physicians practiced in relative isolation, fearful of bringing themselves to the attention of others or expressing opinions that could be interpreted in a political sense. Patients were encouraged to challenge the authority of physicians and to participate in decisions about their own medical care. Our own observations of patient-physician interactions on the ward indicate that this kind of activity is rare when serious medical decisions are involved. (See chapters 7 and 8.) Still, the Cultural Revolution was undeniably a time when the authority and autonomy of physicians were seriously challenged, and the power of physicians and scientists within the unit organizations was undoubtedly at its nadir.

Since the Cultural Revolution, China's emphasis on technical modernization has brought a concomitant rise in the status of its physicians and technical experts. Information is once again at a premium. Advances in medical technology and medical research are valued commodities.[29] There is considerable reliance on technical advisers to the medical college and at the provincial level for information needed to make policy and funding decisions. Even the policies designed to redistribute medical care more evenly throughout the cities and the countryside have taken second place to the modernization effort. Fewer physicians are now assigned to posts in the countryside, and those who are may be increasingly dissatisfied with underutilization of their special skills.

During our stay in China the daily routine on the ward reflected both extensive bureaucratic supervision and considerable physician autonomy in patient care. The physicians reported each contagious disease patient to the provincial disease-prevention station; failure to do so would have resulted in being named as a poor worker in the monthly hospital report. The ward was subject to periodic inspections. Each Saturday morning, everyone joined together to sweep. Political and educational meetings were required. Campaigns were initiated and created more meetings. Models of good and bad performance and behavior were selected by those in authority.

---

deprofessionalize all occupations. In the United States, the goal seems to be to professionalize occupations that suffer potential or actual exploitation by the professions.

29. From the beginning of our experience in the SAH, it was clear that our leaders were eager for us to bring about a demonstrable improvement in the technical capabilities of the hospital. For example, they used our presence as an excuse to convince the provincial authorities to commit funds for the purchase of new machines.

Yet, in areas in which supervision would undermine the power of the physicians in their practice of medicine—that is, in decisions concerning patient care and in relation with the staff who assisted in the delivery of that care—the intrusion of the organization was less evident. Although an atmosphere of comradely egalitarianism characterized interactions on the ward, we never observed a challenge to a physician by the nurses, other medical personnel, or patients. On a daily basis, the physicians were not closely supervised by superiors. On the infectious disease ward, for example, medical rounds with a higher-level physician were conducted only once a week. The fact that physicians were able to exercise control over the practice of medicine despite organizational constraints suggests that their power is indeed derived from control over the information involved in the delivery of medical care (Montagna 1977).

This autonomy does not extend, however, to direct interactions with leaders in supervisory positions. Physicians are deferential to their superiors. On several occasions we observed the physicians responding to the authority of various directors when the latter were present on the ward. This authority relationship has some advantages for physicians. Leaders protect doctors under their jurisdiction and take responsibility for their performance. Reporting a mistake to a leader absolves the physician of responsibility for the error, unless it is very serious. Likewise, a medical-legal dispute that in the United States would be resolved through malpractice litigation, in China is dealt with through negotiation by the work unit leaders of the parties involved.

CAREER MOBILITY

Given the fact that staff are assigned to the *danwei* on a relatively permanent basis, it is clear that the work unit system of job assignment, in combination with other factors, significantly affects career mobility.[30] For professionals and administrators, upward mobility appears to be sporadic and uncertain. A dramatic shift in the criteria used to evaluate performance since the Cultural Revolution is apparent. During the Cultural Revolution, promotions for these occupations ceased. If anything, downward mobility and uncer-

---

30. Several potential influences on career mobility are not discussed here because of the limited data available to us on them. For example, Cole (1979) cites an organization's size as a probable factor in increased mobility. Likewise, it has been suggested that the career mobility described in our unit has occurred in part because Chinese health care facilities have expanded, and with expansion comes upward mobility (Michel Oksenberg, personal communication). Both of these may be important factors, but more comparative data are needed for firm conclusions.

tainty about the future characterized the period. Since then, promotions have resumed and there has been a conscious attempt to reward those who have waited longest. Nevertheless there is a limited number of openings for promotion within any one unit. Another factor constraining upward mobility is the tendency of the *danwei* to "own" its staff. Thus, individuals with opportunities for advancement in other units may be denied such chances by unit leaders who do not want to lose their staff. Furthermore, replacing a professional or administrator often involves replacing a spouse who may want to change jobs and reallocating housing and other services. The unit may also have invested time and money in special training for the staff member, and this investment will be lost if he or she leaves.

The contrast with the permanent employment of professionals and administrators in Japanese companies is striking. There, steady upward mobility is the normal result of working for one firm (Clark 1979, Cole 1979). The Chinese government has recognized the negative impact of unpredictable mobility and frustrated aspirations on Chinese intellectuals and has begun to recommend more flexibility in the work unit system of job assignment and transfer (Hu 1981).

Ironically, these same factors have increased the career mobility of lower-level health personnel. In other countries, these occupations typically promise little upward mobility (Greenfield 1969). In fact, Smith (1955) coined the term *blocked mobility* to describe the limited ladders of advancement available to nurses, medical technicians, physical therapists, respiratory therapists, and other hospital employees in the United States. Blocked career mobility is said to be one of the major factors in job dissatisfaction and in the high turnover of auxiliary employees in hospitals. In these occupations, one of the principal ways of advancing is to leave a job and receive further education or training.

In our hospital unit, the situation was almost reversed. Auxiliary personnel have, for a variety of reasons, experienced far greater career mobility than their American counterparts. Nurses have become doctors, health aides, nurses, and technicians, medical researchers. During different periods, ad hoc systems of promotion have been developed that take into account individual talents and special circumstances. Three major factors seem to explain this phenomenon.

First, the fluidity of job classifications has been largely a product of the radical phases of Chinese politics. For example, the Cultural Revolution's attack on the notion that some people should perform menial work while others carried out "mental" work led to the many changes described earlier.

With the return to job ranks and more standardized methods of job training and advancement, flexibility in promotions will probably decline.

A second explanation for the greater career mobility of lower-level personnel may lie in the fact that medical technology in Chinese hospitals is less sophisticated than in the West. Technology saves labor time and creates new jobs that require a certain level of technical training. Our experience on the infectious disease ward revealed that most of the work of auxiliary personnel is quite labor intensive. Although the hospital is currently emphasizing the need to raise the technical standards of its staff, the skills required to perform most nonphysician tasks are still at a fairly low level. This feature, too, should gradually change as more sophisticated technologies are introduced.

A third factor is the nature of job assignment to work units in China today. Given the circumstances described in earlier chapters, it is not surprising that many units find it easier to retrain existing staff for new jobs or job openings than to attempt to have new staff assigned to the unit. Thus, "internal candidates" have a great advantage. Furthermore, the effort expended by unit leaders to solve some of the employment dilemmas created by the Cultural Revolution, such as the ambiguous position of nurse-doctors, reflects a high level of personal interest in the staff once they belong to the unit. Eventually units will have to resolve the need for additional skilled staff with the lack of a recruiting system, shortage of housing, and the need to provide jobs for spouses.

SUMMARY

Five salient characteristics of work in the *danwei* are: close supervision of the unit's administration and finance by higher levels, and of unit staff by unit leaders; telescoping of party and administrative roles; collective leadership style of decision making; limited exit options for staff; and ritualized participation of the staff in the management of the organization, with indirect mechanisms for expression of staff opinions. These characteristics combine to place a great deal of power in the hands of unit administrators and to produce a specific set of norms of behavior, authority relationships, and career outcomes for unit members. Except in the formal rituals of criticism and consultation, unit staff demonstrate their dependence on the organization by engaging in deferential relationships with unit leaders. These authority relationships, however, mask the indirect methods that staff have developed to deal with conflict and dissatisfaction, namely, expressing opinions through group voice and going around a leader through appeals to higher levels. The unit leaders' passive response to conflict reveals their own dependence on the organization and on higher levels of authority.

Finally, both work autonomy and career mobility of unit members are influenced by the *danwei*. In particular, the combination of no exit, bureaucratic supervision, and the overconcentration of administrative power in party hands places substantial limits on the autonomy of hospital personnel; physicians, however, manage to circumvent these limits to some degree. Career mobility for professionals and administrators has been constrained by the unit system, whereas that of lower-level personnel has been increased.

6

Patients in the *Danwei*

THE REFERRAL SYSTEM

The Second Attached Hospital (SAH) is a tertiary-care facility; that is, it admits patients referred from both primary-care (clinic) and secondary-care (hospital) settings (see figure 8). The SAH also admits patients directly from its own outpatient department. The latter are generally from the immediate vicinity, whereas referral patients may be from anywhere within the hospital's assigned referral zone.

Patients in Wuhan can enter the health services network at a variety of locations, depending on the kind of work unit they belong to, where they live, and how sick they are. The larger work units in China (over 100 staff) usually have clinic facilities on the unit grounds, and members are allowed to go to these clinics when they first become ill. Unless the unit is quite large, the clinic is equipped to treat only minor illness and most of the staff may be paraprofessionals (*yishi*) with only two to three years' training at a technical secondary school. Units with several thousand members and two or three times that number of relatives have medical facilities rivaling those of the local municipal hospitals. The factory down the street from our hospital has health care services typical of a large unit. The factory *danwei* has a population of 40,000. The medical facilities include two infirmaries, each of which treats 20 people per day; an outpatient department similar to the one at the SAH, which sees more than 300 patients per day; a family practice clinic; an obstetrics and gynecology clinic, which keeps detailed records on the fertility and family planning practices of all women in the unit; and a general clinic for on-duty workers. The health personnel at this facility consist of 27 physicians (17 with M.D.s, 10 with lesser degrees), 39 nurses, and

89

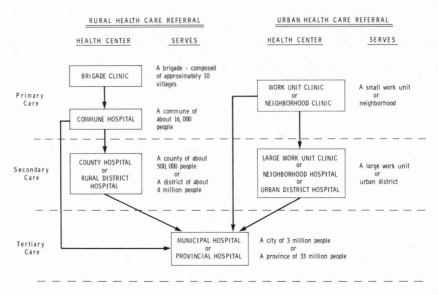

Figure 8. The Patient Referral System

20 other staff. Patients can stay in the outpatient department for several days, but when further care is needed they are referred to a city hospital.

For their first medical visit, patients are free to choose among the many neighborhood health stations and larger clinic facilities scattered throughout the city.[1] These are of varying size and quality. A neighborhood outpatient clinic in Qingdao Shandong Province, described by a recent student tour, saw 100 patients per day, 5 percent of whom were referred to the municipal hospital directly supervising the clinic. Of the twenty-two medical staff assigned to this clinic, ten were physicians ("Health Care and The People's Republic of China" 1979). Victor and Ruth Sidel described a neighborhood hospital in Beijing (visited in the early seventies) as follows:

> This hospital occupies two large courtyards and has seven departments: medicine, surgery, acupuncture, traditional bone medicine, gynecology, dentistry, and tuberculosis; and four auxiliary units: pharmacy (including both traditional Chinese and Western drugs), laboratory, X ray, and

1. The Sidels (1973, 1982) and others make much of the health stations run by the neighborhood residence committees and of their locally recruited staff, who have received very limited training. During the Cultural Revolution there was great emphasis on these health stations, but although they persist today, particularly to carry out sanitation and family planning work, none of the patients we talked to had gone to them.

injections. The public health department serving the neighborhood is located in the hospital, which has no beds; patients requiring hospitalization are sent to the People's Hospital in the West District, several blocks from Fengsheng [the neighborhood's name]. (Sidel and Sidel 1973, 50)[2]

Revisiting this hospital in the late seventies, they found "the number of doctors and nurses . . . increased from 58 to 157, new departments . . . added, including orthopedics, ear-nose-throat, and physical therapy, and facilities now include[d] electrocardiography, electroencephalography, and ultrasound" (Sidel and Sidel 1982, 52). This facility is far more sophisticated than most we saw. Although it could not admit patients for care overnight, some neighborhood clinics in Wuhan also provide infirmary facilities.

Patients who are too sick to remain at the local-level clinics are referred by local medical personnel to a more complex facility. Wuhan, unlike many large urban areas in China, has no intermediate district hospitals, so patients are referred directly to the municipal hospitals (similar in organization to the SAH) or to the hospitals attached to the three medical colleges in the city.[3] To prevent overcrowding at any one hospital, the Bureau of Health assigns local-level clinics and hospitals to one or more referral hospitals. This system is intended to keep a large proportion of patients at the bottom, and less costly, rungs of the referral ladder.[4] In an emergency, however, these rules can be waived and the patient taken to the nearest hospital emergency department.

In the countryside, the referral ladder begins with the brigade paramedic, known as the "barefoot doctor" (*chijiao yisheng*).[5] This individual is recruited from the production brigade, given initial training for three to six

2. This neighborhood hospital was probably a "model" hospital, that is, much better than the norm. Furthermore, the high number of M.D.'s was probably a reflection of its location in Beijing.

3. Wuhan, with a population of 3 million, has approximately twelve municipal hospitals and an equal number of specialty hospitals (infectious disease, tuberculosis, children's, and so on).

4. The cost of services at dispensaries or rural health centers in other developing nations has been shown to be six to eight times less than at major referral hospitals like the SAH (Gish 1975, 58).

5. Barefoot doctors were the subject of great interest to foreign visitors studying China's rural health care reforms during the Cultural Revolution (Sidel 1972). Indeed, many have asserted that the new trend in paraprofessionals in the United States (the physician's assistant, the nurse-practitioner) is a result of the influence of China's health care policies. Recently, however, there has been a reported decline in emphasis on barefoot doctors (Lampton 1981, Sidel and Sidel 1982). For detailed descriptions of the work of barefoot doctors, see also Lee (1981).

months followed by periodic continuing education courses, and paid through the same collective workpoint system as fellow brigade members. Almost every brigade in China has at least one barefoot doctor, some have many more. In 1974, the ratio of barefoot doctors to the population was reported at 1:760, in contrast to the pre-Cultural Revolution ratio of 1:8,000 in rural areas (Hu 1975, 10). Today the skill, training, and facilities of the barefoot doctors vary enormously depending on the wealth of the region, and efforts are under way to upgrade and standardize their skills (Sidel and Sidel 1982). We visited a commune on the outskirts of Wuhan that seemed fairly well off, with 30,000 members (6,800 households), 18 brigades (each with its own health station), and 160 production teams. We were taken to a brigade health station (*yiliao suo*) in a brand-new brigade government building. There, five barefoot doctors, each trained for approximately six months at the commune hospital, saw patients for seven or eight months and worked in the fields the rest of the year. They were responsible for the 2,800 people in the brigade (thus the barefoot doctor–population ratio was 1:560) and saw approximately 35 patients per day. Their health station consisted of an office, a small pharmacy with mostly traditional herbs, an injection room, and an examination room. The office was equipped with a desk and chair. The examination room had a narrow cot. The barefoot doctors treated minor cuts, colds, and chronic illness with Western and traditional Chinese medicines and injections. They also conducted family planning, sanitation, and other disease prevention work. Patients who were seriously ill and/or needed to be in an infirmary overnight were referred to the commune hospital outpatient department.

The commune medical facilities were a simplified version of an urban hospital, with eighty staff members (including forty nurses and physicians); outpatient and inpatient departments for internal medicine, surgery, and a few specialties such as pediatrics, and obstetrics and gynecology; and a seventy-five-bed hospital ward. The surgery department could perform operations such as cholecystectomies, appendectomies, and tubal ligations. Serious cases were referred to county hospitals or the higher-level rural district hospitals, which were said to be equivalent in quality to the municipal hospitals in Wuhan. Ultimate referral was to one of the teaching hospitals, which occupy a slightly higher position in the system.[6]

6. The relationship between the city hospitals and the hospitals attached to the medical colleges is hierarchical in only a limited sense. All are referral centers, but when a difficult patient is admitted, the city hospitals will consult with the teaching hospitals. The hospitals attached to Wuhan Medical College, a nationally administered medical college, are thought to be slightly superior to the provincial-level ones such as the SAH.

In Hubei Province, eight districts comprising seventy-two counties refer patients to the urban hospitals in Wuhan. Each of the five teaching hospitals attached to the three medical colleges and some of the more sophisticated municipal hospitals are assigned as referral centers for certain counties and districts. These rural areas also receive the medical personnel sent down from the referral hospitals. The SAH has fifteen referral counties, located in the eastern part of the province within approximately 150 kilometers of Wuhan. It also receives patients from the urban district in which it is located. This district includes neighborhoods as well as work units.

HEALTH INSURANCE

In China, health insurance coverage varies by occupation. Workers in state-owned and some large, collectively owned enterprises receive complete medical coverage from their work units.[7] Workers' dependents are generally provided with coverage for half their medical costs. Cadres in state enterprises (schools, hospitals, factories, government organizations, and other state-owned businesses) are also offered complete medical coverage. Generally the dependents of cadres are not given insurance benefits, although local-level units such as Hubei Provincial Medical College may decide to offer an insurance program funded by a monthly premium payment (at HPMC it is one yuan per month per child). Under these health insurance programs, the reimbursement mechanism is also intended to serve as an incentive for patients to comply with the official referral policies. Patients must go first to the designated work unit or neighborhood health clinic, and referral to a higher-level facility occurs with only the recommendation of the local-level physician or paramedic. A referral reimbursement form (*sanliandan*) is given to the patient to present at the appropriate hospital accounting department; this form is sent, after the patient is discharged, to the patient's *danwei* for payment. Without this form, the patient is liable for payment unless the illness was clearly a medical emergency.

Peasants and temporary workers with household registrations in the communes are insured through a variety of cooperative insurance programs. The cost to the peasant, the contribution of the collective, and the extent of coverage depend completely on the sale of the commune's agricultural crops and the output of its light industries. At the commune we visited, the peas-

7. The so-called complete coverage does not include food (which in the SAH averaged .5 yuan a day); the .05-yuan registration fee; unusually costly medicines; and items such as eyeglasses, crutches, or dentures.

ants reportedly paid one yuan per person per year for medical insurance; the commune and the production team each contributed two yuan per person per year for the collective medical insurance fund. This system, we were told, provided complete coverage for the peasants in the commune. Other peasants are not so fortunate. As Blendon has noted, "With the financing of health services left to the capacity of each co-operative, serious imbalances occur" (1979, 1454). Indeed, communes that cannot afford to offer complete health insurance coverage—and these are undoubtedly the majority— provide either a percentage of total costs or a fixed amount of medical expenses, with the peasants liable for the remainder.[8] Several peasants on the infectious disease ward reported that although they paid one to two yuan per person per year for insurance, they were still responsible for about 30 percent of their bills.

The system of reimbursement for peasants also differs from that for workers and cadres. When peasants become ill and need medical care, they must pay the cost themselves before they leave the hospital, and then submit the bill for reimbursement. At the SAH, peasants must put down a deposit on their bill before they are admitted, unless the case is an emergency (100 yuan for surgery patients and 80 yuan for internal medicine patients).[9] Thus, whereas referral regulations operate to restrain urban residents from overutilizing the more sophisticated health care facilities, the initial cost of utilization and distance from the hospital stem the tide of peasants into city hospitals.[10]

Health insurance coverage for workers in most collectively owned enterprises is similar to that for peasants; each collective runs its own insurance program. Workers are rarely provided with complete coverage and dependents may not be covered at all. As in the countryside, the extent of insurance depends on how successful the enterprise is. Furthermore, workers who have been ill pay for their medical expenses first and obtain reimbursement later for some proportion from their work units.[11]

8. The fixed-amount coverage in poor brigades may be about 50 yuan per person per year, in rich brigades 100–200 yuan per person per year (Martin K. Whyte, personal communication).

9. Presumably this deposit is required because the peasants and their rural cooperatives occasionally renege on their debts.

10. Apparently peasants are sometimes able to come to urban referral hospitals without going through all the referral levels. Near Beijing, for example, peasants in suburban brigades close to a city hospital often simply come with a letter from a barefoot doctor (Martin K. Whyte, personal communication).

11. Information regarding insurance for workers in collective enterprises was provided by Martin K. Whyte (personal communication).

PATIENTS ADMITTED TO THE
SAH INFECTIOUS DISEASE WARD

To understand better how the referral system works and how individuals make greatest use of their health care services (discussed in chapter 7), we studied the medical records of eighty-four patients admitted to the infectious disease ward from December 1979 to March 1980.[12] With the help of the ward staff, we recorded the following variables for eighty-two cases: residence and distance from the SAH, occupation, diagnosis, degree of seriousness of illness, length of stay, and type of insurance coverage. Interviews with seventy-six patients provided detailed information about access routes to the SAH, including referrals from lower-level or intermediate health care facilities and other, nonstandard routes of admission. (The remaining six patients were not on the ward long enough, were too ill to be interviewed, or were children.) From the SAH accounting department we obtained the inpatient cost of nineteen patients, selected on the basis of type and severity of illness.[13]

The SAH has a potential referral population of approximately 750,000 urban residents and about 7 million rural residents. Despite this predominately rural population, the majority of patients (72 percent) admitted to the infectious disease ward during the study were from Wuhan and suburban areas. This figure includes fifty-one urban residents, four peasants from a suburban commune, and four peasants on temporary work assignment in the city. The remaining 28 percent were from prescribed referral counties, ranging from 50 to 150 kilometers from the hospital (see figure 9). Of all the patients studied, 94 percent were from the appropriate referral regions. Only five patients were from nonreferral counties, ranging from 50 to 600 kilometers away. These patients were either hospitalized while traveling through Wuhan or were transferred to the SAH for specialized care not available in their own referral hospital.

The twenty-three patients who were referred from rural counties had traveled a considerable distance to reach the SAH. Roughly half had trav-

12. Detailed analysis of the results is available in Henderson and Cohen (1982).

13. Clearly, the best method to evaluate the efficacy of the referral system would have been to begin with the total potentially ill population—that is, to have surveyed first all people in the SAH's fifteen counties and urban referral areas who were ill during this period, then those who were admitted to the SAH, and finally to have compared their characteristics with those of all the people who were ill. Unfortunately, it was impossible to conduct such a survey at that time. Consequently, our conclusions about the nature of access to a facility such as the SAH are at best tentative.

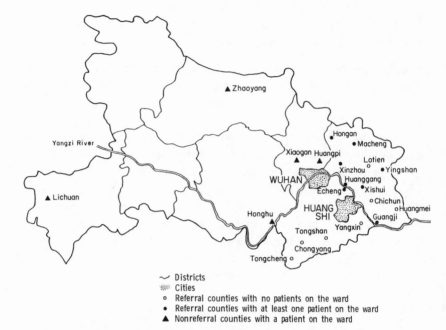

~ Districts
 ⁂ Cities
 ○ Referral counties with no patients on the ward
 • Referral counties with at least one patient on the ward
 ▲ Nonreferral counties with a patient on the ward

Figure 9. Rural Referrals to the Second Attached Hospital's Infectious Disease
Ward, December 1979–March 1980, Hubei Province

eled more than 75 kilometers, and 26 percent of these more than 100 kilometers (equivalent to a day's bus or boat ride). As might be expected, more referrals came from nearby than from distant counties. Eight of the fifteen
referral counties were represented on the ward, and there was at least one
patient from each of the five referral counties less than 100 kilometers from
the hospital. Only three of the ten counties located more than 100 kilometers away were represented.

All patients at the SAH are ranked according to severity of illness,
based on the level of nursing care required.[14] Sixty-three percent of the patients in the infectious disease ward were classified as mild, 22 percent as serious, and 15 percent as critical. At a high-level referral hospital, where one
expects the majority of patients to be quite sick, we found this distribution

14. In the infectious disease ward, these three gradations were carefully recorded at the
nursing station each day. On a wooden chart listing all the ward beds, each patient was
awarded no marker, a blue marker, or a red marker. No marker indicated that the patient could
walk about and feed himself or herself; red, that all nursing tasks must be done by the nurses;
blue, that the patient would be helped as much as needed.

surprising. Severity of illness was highly related to location: 85 percent of the mildly ill patients were from the city, whereas only slightly more than half of the more seriously ill patients were urban residents.

The explanation for these distributions lies, in part, in the government's infectious disease regulations. Patients with hepatitis must be admitted to a hospital ward. Because many hepatitis patients are only mildly ill, the city hospitals accommodate urban hepatitis patients, whereas the rural hepatitis patients are generally not sick enough to warrant transfer from hospitals in the countryside. Furthermore, hepatitis may be more common in the cities than in the countryside. Fifty-nine percent of the patients on the infectious disease ward suffered from hepatitis.

Given that patients admitted to the infectious disease ward are more likely to live in the city, it is also not surprising that the patient population was composed primarily of workers and cadres. Thirty-three percent of the patients were workers, 34 percent were cadres, and 7 percent were dependents of workers and cadres. Only 26 percent were peasants (farmers) and 1 percent state farm workers.

As was mentioned earlier, insurance coverage for patients varies according to occupation. In our study, 67 percent of the patients on the infectious disease ward—including the state farm worker, who was considered an employee in a state enterprise—were fully covered by their work units for their hospitalization costs. Thirty-three percent had only partial coverage.

PATIENT CHARGES

Many visitors to China have described its medical care as remarkably inexpensive (Sidel and Sidel 1973, Hu 1975, Cheng 1973).[15] Our study of patient costs in a tertiary-care facility yields the opposite conclusion. Table 1 summarizes the cost of hospitalization for nineteen patients selected to reflect the spectrum of diseases admitted to the ward. The average cost per day to all nineteen patients was 5.34 yuan ($3.56). Food costs, paid separately, totaled approximately .5 yuan ($.33) per day.[16] For these patients, medicine

15. Hu stated that a commune member pays "only a minimal amount of money for the treatment and medicines he receives" and that "expense isn't a barrier to medical care" (1975, 22). According to Cheng, "Medical care . . . is free . . . or costs very little. . . " (1973, 286). On the other hand, Blendon (1979) and other more recent observers have pointed out that medical costs *can* be high. And even as early as 1974, Lampton clearly identified the disadvantage of the peasant with less income and less health care coverage.

16. The prices of a typical sample of meals from the patients' kitchen, in yuan and U.S. dollars, are as follows: cabbage, .06 ($.04); pork and egg, .35 ($.24); fatty pork and onions, .25 ($.17); sour beans and pork, .20 ($.14); and *caitai* (a Hubei vegetable), .10 ($.07).

Table 1. Costs of Hospitalization for Nineteen Infectious Disease Patients, in Yuan and U.S. Dollars

Disease	Average Daily Patient Charge	Average Total Patient Charge	Average Total Patient Charge, Including Food
Schistosomiasis (N = 3)	2.24 ± 2.72($1.49 ± 1.81)	87.00 ($58.00)	106.31 ($70.87)
Hepatitis (N = 6)	8.04 ± 3.54($5.36 ± 2.36)	225.00 ($150.00)	238.86 ($159.24)
Epidemic hemorrhagic fever (N = 3)	6.09 ± 3.15($4.06 ± 2.10)	267.96 ($178.64)	289.74 ($193.16)
Dysentery (N = 4)	2.60 ± .51($1.73 ± .34)	76.55 ($51.03)	91.16 ($60.77)
Fever of unknown origin (N = 3)	6.00 ± 1.65($4.00 ± 1.10)	82.20 ($54.80)	88.98 ($59.32)

Note: The exchange rate used is $1.00 U.S. = 1.50 yuan.
Note: ± = standard deviation.

accounted for 42.6 percent of costs, room 23.9 percent, treatment 17.1 percent, laboratory tests 6.7 percent, heat 5.8 percent, and X rays 4.7 percent. Had this been a surgical ward, treatment costs would have represented a larger part of the bill and probably increased the total cost dramatically. Furthermore, although inpatient costs at a tertiary facility such as the SAH exceed those at a lower-level hospital, the costs discussed here are only a portion of the total cost of hospitalization: staff salaries, administrative fees, hospital maintainance, and capital investment costs are not represented in the patient's bill but are covered under the state budget. Table 2 presents a breakdown of costs for the nineteen patients on our ward and for patients at the North Carolina Memorial Hospital, adjusted to permit comparison.[17]

17. Comparative data on the breakdown of patient bills in the United States are difficult to obtain. Although the North Carolina Memorial Hospital, like the SAH, is a state-run referral center that also serves as a teaching hospital for a major medical school and is similar in size (572 beds) and in number of outpatients, the number of inpatients is more than twice as large because of their considerably shorter length of stay (19 versus 8.9 days). Data provided by Bill J. Fuller, Associate Director of Fiscal Services at NCMH, are for all patients admitted in fiscal 1980; specific data on the bills of infectious disease patients were not available. The NCMH breakdown is as follows: pharmacy (including IV), 13.8 percent; laboratory (including pathology and blood bank), 16.1 percent; radiology, 8.3 percent; room and board (including nurses'

Table 2. Breakdown of Patient Costs at the Second Attached Hospital and
North Carolina Memorial Hospital, Adjusted for Comparison

	NCMH	SAH
Pharmacy	25%	51%
Laboratory	29	8
Radiology	15	6
Room, board, and heat	31	35

Note: There is far less use of diagnostic testing in China than in the United States. See chapter 8 for discussion.

Source: NCMH data are from Bill J. Fuller, Associate Director of Fiscal Services, North Carolina Memorial Hospital, Chapel Hill (personal communication).

Even with the state absorbing much of the actual cost, the bills (paid in full by the work units, or in part by the rural or urban collective insurance programs) can be substantial. For the selected patients in the five disease categories treated on the infectious disease ward, average total costs ranged from 88.98 yuan ($59.32) for fever of unknown origin to 289.74 yuan ($193.16) for epidemic hemorrhagic fever. The range of all nineteen patient bills was 10.70 yuan ($7.13) plus food for a dysentery patient who stayed only six days, to 508.03 yuan ($338.69) plus food for a patient with epidemic hemorrhagic fever who was hospitalized for forty-one days. The average total charge to all patients studied was 178.29 yuan ($118.86).

These figures are best understood in terms of per-capita income in

---

salaries [over 50 percent], utilities, overhead, other staff salaries except M.D.s, equipment assigned to a particular ward—amortized over several years—and food), 35.8 percent; surgery (including operating, recovery, and delivery rooms; anesthesiology; occupational therapy; and physical therapy), 12.1 percent; and other costs (including emergency room, outpatient clinics, and supplies), 13.9 percent.

One major element not included in patients' bills at NCMH is physicians' salaries and charges for physicians' procedures. Those fees are charged to the patient separately and paid to the medical school that staffs the hospital. All other staff salaries come out of the room and board charge to patients, the greatest proportion going to nurses' salaries. At the SAH, no staff salaries are included in patients' bills, except the part of the room charge going to nursing care (which may be translated into nurses' salaries at the provincial level but does not transfer directly). The treatment charge at the SAH is for physicians' procedures.

To obtain a comparable breakdown of patient costs for the nineteen patients on the infectious disease ward and patients at NCMH, then, we must eliminate the treatment figure for the SAH and, for NCMH, the figures for surgery, other costs, and half the room and board costs (to account for nurses' salaries and for food costs).

China. The average yearly income for all hospital staff in our *danwei* was approximately 756 yuan, ranging from 420 to 2,400 yuan. Recent Chinese publications have reported the annual per-capita income for state-sector employees in 1979 as 704 yuan (Zhou 1980) and for Shanghai and surrounding counties (China's wealthiest region) as 1,600 yuan (*Beijing Review* 24, no. 37 [14 September 1981]: 3). For peasants, especially those living in poorer regions, income is considerably lower. According to Chinese sources, the entire annual income for all peasants in 1977 was 117 yuan; in 1980, 170 yuan (*Beijing Review* 24, no. 39 [28 September 1981]: 3). These figures underestimate actual peasant per-capita income because they average all rural people together (including many nonproductive family members). Nevertheless, recent research has concluded that the income of urban Chinese is probably three times that of rural Chinese (Parish 1981).[18] This means that those who can least afford it are personally liable for the greatest portion of their hospital bills, whereas those who earn the most are not required to pay anything except food costs and special fees. The peasant on our ward who had a hospital bill of 508 yuan reported that he belonged to a collective insurance program that provided 70 percent coverage. He was thus responsible for 152.41 yuan, probably equivalent to more than half a year's income.

The physicians on the infectious disease ward were conscious of the cost of hospitalization to patients. They indicated that cost containment sometimes played a role in their choice of medication for peasants and in their decision to discharge certain patients who could not benefit from care.[19] On the other hand, several infectious and other diseases that are endemic to the countryside—including malaria, schistosomiasis, and brucellosis—are treated free of charge. Patients pay for their care but are reimbursed by the local governments.

PATIENT REFERRAL STRATEGIES

In our investigation of the referral routes to the outpatient department and to the infectious disease ward, we found that city dwellers used the facilities of the outpatient department far more extensively than did peasants. Despite strict regulations prohibiting referral to the SAH without a recom-

18. Recent Chinese surveys indicate that urban families have about four members and that about 55 percent of the urban population is employed. Thus, on a per-capita basis (parallel to the rural figures) 1979 urban income would have been about 387 yuan, or about three times the 1979 rural income estimates (Martin K. Whyte, personal communication).

19. For example, physicians delayed a blood transfusion for a peasant until his son arrived to pay for it (40 yuan per 100 cc of blood) and it became clear that he really needed it. Had he been in great need, they said, they would have given it without considering the cost.

mendation (and the requirement for a reimbursement form from lower-level facilities), the same number of patients were observed going directly to the SAH outpatient department as to the appropriate *danwei* or neighborhood clinic. A few of these were in fact unable to go to the lower-level clinics because of the time at which their illness occurred or its critical nature. Yet most of the patients interviewed stated that they knew they could obtain the referral form *after* their visit; and indeed, on many of the worker and cadre charts we reviewed, the coverage was listed as "self-pay" (*zifei*) instead of the expected "charge to the account" (*jizhang*) that should accompany those possessing insurance. The staff at the nursing station explained that even though these patients had failed to obtain the reimbursement form beforehand, they would surely receive coverage. The staff found this strategy neither unusual nor surprising. As we got acquainted with the ward and the patients we realized that people in Wuhan use the hospital outpatient and emergency departments in much the same way Americans do. Patients visit local clinics for the sake of convenience, for minor illnesses; however, for any illness they believe to be serious, they frequently bypass the designated access route. The statistics on the enormous number of patients seen in the outpatient departments of the First and Second Attached Hospitals (1,000 and 1,500 per day, respectively) are testimony to this phenomenon.

In addition, physicians on the infectious disease ward occasionally remarked on urban patients' reluctance to depend on the lower-level health personnel. One noted that the outpatient departments are crowded with patients whose illnesses could easily be dealt with at unit or neighborhood clinics, and that even when patients go first to those clinics, they are reluctant to wait to see if the therapy prescribed will work. Instead, they persuade the clinic staff to refer them to higher levels or go directly from the smaller clinics to the outpatient departments for further examination. Some lower-level medical personnel act to prevent this easy upward flow, and the frequent lack of available beds in tertiary-care facilities also serves to limit upward referral. Still, it appears that the referral system, whose aim is to weed out all but the sickest before they are referred to higher, more expensive levels, may not be as efficient as intended.[20]

For those in the countryside, particularly the peasants who live a fair

20. Since we left China, it appears that local-level units, under pressure from the recent campaigns to economize, have cracked down on the laxness of the referral system. Reports indicate that it is not quite so easy to go to the SAH without a referral and that the units are keeping close (and public) track of how much each staff member is costing in terms of insurance coverage.

distance from Wuhan, the system seems to be functioning more smoothly.[21] The peasants and rural cadres on our ward tended to follow the prescribed access routes, beginning at the commune level. Those peasants who did follow an urban route either were temporary workers already in the city or had some personal connections there.

Our observations and interviews with outpatients revealed that, regardless of the large number of regulations to control their movements, patients have a fair amount of flexibility in the system, especially if they are willing to pay for health care out of their own pockets. We characterized the nonstandard admissions to the infectious disease ward, which accounted for 26 percent of the patients we studied. Six patients (two cadres, two peasants, and two dependents) initiated referral to be closer to a relative. It is common for parents, such as those of the two children on our ward, to request that their children be placed in hospitals close to their place of work, even if it is not the correct referral hospital. Another city patient on our ward had first been placed in a hospital close to his work unit but not to his home, and because he wanted his wife to be able to see him, he requested transfer to the SAH. The other referrals were from the countryside and they felt more comfortable being admitted to a hospital near some urban relative who could look after them.

Fifteen patients (five workers, seven cadres, and three peasants) initiated referral to the SAH because they felt it was a better hospital than their designated referral hospital. Among these, the following four cases were typical.

A thirty-eight-year-old male doing temporary food transport work near Wuhan and originally from Xiaogan County, 100 kilometers away, became ill with viral hepatitis and went to the nearest outpatient department, at Wuhan City Hospital 7 in Wuchang. He was admitted and chose the department of combined Western and Chinese traditional medicine. After two months he felt there was no improvement, so he left the hospital and came to the SAH outpatient department because it had "better equipment." Because there were no beds in the infectious disease ward, he waited three days in his unit's clinic before being admitted. He stayed more than seventy days.

A twenty-nine-year-old female worker in the Wuhan Watch Factory

21. There is little doubt that the readiness with which urban residents availed themselves of the SAH outpatient department is mirrored in the countryside in commune hospitals and county and district hospitals. Patients will always tend to make such use of nearby outpatient departments.

who lived in the factory housing down the road from the SAH became ill with viral hepatitis and went to her factory clinic. She was diagnosed as having "aching nerves" and was treated with vitamins. Because a friend had noticed that her eyeballs were yellow, the patient asked a physician friend in the SAH internal medicine department to arrange an examination. This physician took her to the SAH outpatient department, but when tests were negative, he arranged further examination in the internal medicine laboratory. The patient was ultimately admitted to the infectious disease ward with hepatitis, where she stayed for thirty-seven days.

A twenty-nine-year-old female peasant from a commune in Xinzhou County, about 50 kilometers from the SAH, became ill and went to the commune clinic, where she received traditional medicine. She was subsequently admitted to the commune hospital with a diagnosis of a necrotic liver. During the month she was there, she received both traditional and Western medicine. Twenty days after being discharged from the commune hospital, she developed ascites (serous fluid in the stomach). Relatives working at Wuhan City Hospital 3 (affiliated with Wuhan Medical College, the national-level college) urged her to avail herself of better care at their hospital, so she went to the outpatient department there. She was examined and released twice. On her third trip to Wuhan, she went to another hospital affiliated with Wuhan Medical College. There she was given traditional medicine and returned home yet again. She then came to the SAH outpatient department and was admitted to the infectious disease ward with a tentative diagnosis of hepatitis or cirrhosis. She stayed more than two months.

A thirty-seven-year-old female cadre in the Bureau of Machinery of Hubei Province, in Wuchang, contracted hepatitis for a second time. She chose the outpatient department of the affiliated hospital of Wuhan's Chinese Traditional Medicine College because she had heard that the physicians there were investigating hepatitis B. She took traditional medicine but after suffering acute gastrointestinal discomfort went to the SAH outpatient department. She was treated there for one day, went home for three, and after jaundice developed was admitted to the infectious disease ward, where she stayed more than fifty days.

From these brief histories, it is clear that patients feel quite comfortable about going to various outpatient departments if they suspect their treatment can be improved. Flagrant doctor-shopping, however, was uncommon enough to warrant special mention by the physicians on our ward. In only two of the twenty-one nonstandard referrals did patients visit five or more hospitals before arriving on our ward. In one of these cases, there was a lack of available beds; in the other, the patient was dissatisfied with the care or diagnosis received. Initiation of referral did not seem to be related to where patients lived or worked.

As indicated above, the majority of patients admitted to the infectious disease ward were from the city, whereas only 28 percent were referred from rural counties. In comparison with other developing countries, the percentage of rural referrals is impressive. Surveys in Africa, for example, have shown that less than 10 percent of inpatients in national referral hospitals similar to the SAH can be expected to come from outside the city (Gish 1975, 46). On the other hand, statistics from the North Carolina Memorial Hospital, a teaching hospital at a major medical center that admits patients referred from an entire state (with a population comparable to that of Wuhan itself), show that only 17.9 percent of inpatients are from the county in which the hospital is located. The remainder (79.3 percent) have been referred from elsewhere in the state and from outside the state (2.8 percent).[22]

CASE STUDIES OF PATIENT REFERRAL

The following case studies highlight the diversity of patient strategies and care on the infectious disease ward.[23]

Case 1

A twenty-six-year-old female with no prior illness was employed as a middle school mathematics teacher in Wuchang, not far from the SAH. On 27 October 1979, she visited the middle school clinic complaining of stomach pains and was examined by a paramedic, who sent her home to rest. Over the next three days she developed arthritis and went to the neighborhood street hospital (*jiedao yiyuan*) appropriate for her housing residence. At this clinic she was examined by a physician and a diagnosis of rheumatism was made. She was admitted to the hospital's ten-bed facility the next day and was treated with an antimicrobial agent. Her symptoms persisted over the next two weeks and she became dissatisfied with her progress and left this

---

22. Bill J. Fuller, Associate Director of Fiscal Services, North Carolina Memorial Hospital (personal communication).

23. These three case reports appear in Henderson and Cohen (1982).

hospital. At the suggestion of a friend, she went to the outpatient department of the SAH (without informing them of her admission to the neighborhood hospital), where liver function tests revealed acute hepatitis. She then returned to the street hospital with this information and received therapy appropriate for hepatitis. Over the next two weeks, she failed to improve but the street hospital physician refused to allow transfer to another hospital, and she returned home.

She remained at home for approximately ten days. During this time she was treated with herbal medicine administered by a neighbor who was self-taught in Chinese traditional medicine. Although her systemic symptoms improved slightly, she developed jaundice and went to the outpatient department of the hospital attached to the Chinese Traditional Medicine College in Wuhan. There, hepatitis was again diagnosed, but she was not admitted because of lack of available beds. After returning home briefly, she requested admission to the First Attached Hospital of Hubei Provincial Medical College, but no beds were available on their infectious disease ward. She visited her work unit leader for advice and was subsequently admitted to the infectious disease ward of the SAH. She remained hospitalized for forty-one days until her jaundice had disappeared and was discharged 24 January 1980. Her hospitalization was paid by her work unit under the cadre medical insurance program. The hospital bill is as follows:

Room	28.70 yuan ($19.13)
Heat	8.20 yuan ($5.47)
Medicine	57.62 yuan ($38.41)
Procedures	31.60 yuan ($21.07)
Laboratories	8.80 yuan ($5.87)
X rays	4.00 yuan ($2.67)
Subtotal	138.92 yuan ($92.62)
Food	20.50 yuan ($13.67)
Total	159.42 yuan ($106.29)

This case illustrates the wide variety of options available to the Chinese patient. The young woman was dissatisfied with the care she was receiving at the first level to which she was referred—the neighborhood hospital outpatient department—and she subsequently referred herself to several other outpatient departments. She also took advantage of Chinese traditional medicine, which many Chinese patients feel is most appropriate for chronic illness. It is surprising that she was not immediately admitted to an infectious disease ward when the diagnosis of hepatitis was made, for government rules require that patients with this illness remain hospitalized in isolation until jaundice disappears. The lack of available beds for admission to higher-level hospitals like the SAH, however, is a common complaint. Although it is unclear how important a role this young woman's *danwei* leader played in her ultimate admission to the infectious disease ward at the SAH, her visit to her unit leader is consistent with the approach to health care taken by several patients interviewed. (The role of unit leaders in health care is discussed further in chapter 7.) The patient's hospital costs were typical for hepatitis.

Case 2

A fifty-six-year-old male peasant with no prior illness lived in a commune approximately sixty kilometers from the SAH. On 24 November 1979, he developed fever, headache, and a variety of other systemic symptoms. He was examined at the brigade clinic on the same day by a barefoot doctor and was treated for fever, but failed to improve. On the morning of 26 November he was referred to the commune hospital for further evaluation. The physical exam revealed hypotension (low blood pressure) and other symptoms consistent with epidemic hemorrhagic fever. That evening he was transferred to the SAH, the referral center for his commune. The county hospital was bypassed for unknown reasons. He remained on the infectious disease ward for forty-one days and received supportive therapy until 6 January 1980. The breakdown of expenses during his hospitalization is as follows:

Room	28.70 yuan ($19.13)
Heat	7.00 yuan ($4.67)
Medicine	209.23 yuan ($139.49)
Blood	190.90 yuan ($127.27)
Oxygen	2.40 yuan ($1.60)
Procedures	27.40 yuan ($18.27)
Laboratories	42.20 yuan ($28.13)
Room charges for relative	.20 yuan ($.13)
Subtotal	508.03 yuan ($338.69)
Food	20.50 yuan ($13.67)
Total	528.53 yuan ($352.36)

This man followed the guidelines of the health care referral system. As soon as he became ill, he was seen and examined by paramedical personnel, and within a brief time, when it was obvious that he was too sick for brigade clinic care, he was transferred to the commune clinic. Epidemic hemorrhagic fever has such a high morbidity and mortality rate (Cohen et al. 1981, Cohen 1982) that patients with this disease are rapidly transferred to tertiary-care facilities. This fact may explain why he was not transferred to the county or district hospital from the commune clinic. In addition, his commune is less than half a day's journey from Wuhan by car. Had he lived much farther away, he might have been referred initially to a rural referral center. During his hospitalization at the SAH, he received only symptomatic therapy and blood transfusions. Blood is expensive in China—(40 yuan ($26.67) for 100 cc. Under his collective's insurance program, the patient will be required to pay approximately 30 percent of his total bill.

Case 3

A twenty-three-year-old male peasant living in Yingshan County, about 150 kilometers from the SAH, was well until 22 February 1980, when he developed systemic symptoms and a diagnosis of viral hepatitis was made. When his condition worsened, he was transferred by bus from local facilities to the SAH. There his condition deteriorated further and he developed coma and bleeding. Because of a local belief that marriage will bring a sick person luck, while the young man was still in the hospital his sister dressed up in man's clothes and was "married" to his girl friend in a ceremony on the commune grounds. Nevertheless, he continued to deteriorate. At that point the physicians on the ward discussed the possibility of further hospitalization, blood transfusions, and nonspecific supportive therapy. Because the doctors suggested that there was little hope for survival and the cost of hospitalization would be high, the patient's family removed him from the hospital and he returned on 4 March 1980 to his local commune, where he died. Hospital charges for this patient were not available for review.

This patient is typical of many we evaluated, for whom the cost of hospitalization was an overriding concern.

SUMMARY AND IMPLICATIONS FOR UTILIZATION AND COST

Almost all the patients studied on the infectious disease ward were admitted to hospitals in their assigned referral area. The routes of referral, however, varied. It appears that the shorter and more flexible urban route results in the admission of more urban workers and cadres than of rural peasants and cadres and, furthermore, that urban patients are admitted for less serious illness than are rural patients. One explanation is the impact of the national health regulations regarding hepatitis.[24] Another is the difficulty of travel and the opportunity costs involved for the peasant who is referred to a city hospital.[25] Finally, and probably most important, the quality of health care services available to peasants in the countryside at the county and district hospitals has improved dramatically in the past three decades. Thus in a large number of cases, referral to a tertiary-care facility may not be necessary. One physician on the infectious disease ward who had come back from countryside duty commented that many county hospitals in the rural areas of Hubei Province could handle most of the patients seen at the SAH. On the other hand, few commune hospitals are equivalent in quality to the one at the SAH. Furthermore, peasants pay more for health care than do most urban residents. Studies elsewhere have demonstrated a clear relationship between amount of insurance coverage and rate of utilization of services (Aday and Anderson 1978).

Our results suggest that the two most effective ways to reduce the cost of tertiary health care in China would be to alter both patient health care behavior and physician prescribing habits (that is, to avoid use of medications that have no documented benefit). These recommendations may be difficult to implement. First, as in other socialist medical care settings in which the state employs the physician on a fixed salary (and controls other income-generating facilities), there are no incentives to the physician for early discharge of patients. Second, because the vast majority of urban residents are in the labor force, it is impractical to expect a family member to stay at home with a convalescing patient. Third, patient and family expectations are directed toward therapy, even for diseases for which therapy offers little benefit. This is a crucial factor in cost containment because in China, as in many other developing countries, therapy represents the major expense in health care costs (Henderson and Cohen 1982). In addition, several government rules enforce prolonged hospitalization. Patients with hepatitis (a very common disease in China), for example, must remain in the hospital until they are no longer jaundiced, even though the period of contagion may be much shorter. Reducing the use of medications involves changing patient expectations and physician prescribing habits; both tasks will be exceedingly difficult.

24. The other diseases seen on the infectious disease ward are also related to geography. Dysentery is a short-lived disease process that is likely to improve before transfer becomes necessary. Epidemic hemorrhagic fever, however, is limited to areas in the countryside where the mouse vector is ubiquitous (Henderson and Cohen 1982).

25. These opportunity costs involve the expense of travel, the loss of workpoints and other income from one's job in the countryside, and the financial losses of relatives accompanying the patient. (Workers and cadres have sick leaves; peasants do not.)

On the other hand, China's tremendous success in the use of political solutions to social problems deserves emphasis. In this regard, administrative solutions that take advantage of the work units' control over personnel and clients may be effective in changing the distribution and cost of health care. The recent drive to economize (which has received a great deal of attention in Chinese hospitals) may make urban work unit leaders more conscious of the health insurance costs that workers and cadres accumulate.[26] Strict adherence to rules that impede unnecessary referral to higher-level, more expensive hospitals such as our unit would effectively reduce costs. Work units and urban neighborhoods may also be mobilized to provide volunteers to care for recuperating patients, and thus reduce hospitalization.

Perhaps most important, upgrading technology and the quality of care in county and commune hospitals has had a major impact on health care and is more cost effective and easier to implement than trying to reduce costs in tertiary-care facilities. Upgrading the rural health care system (giving "shoes" to barefoot doctors) is also a clear message in favor of distribution of excellent health care services to the massive rural population (Wu 1981).

26. The economic program is called the "Five Settlements": (1) set your tasks, (2) set your number of beds, (3) set your ratio of beds to staff at 1.7 to 1 (quite far from the actual ratio at our hospital), (4) set competence levels for staff (through examinations), and (5) set amount of money for each hospital's deficit.

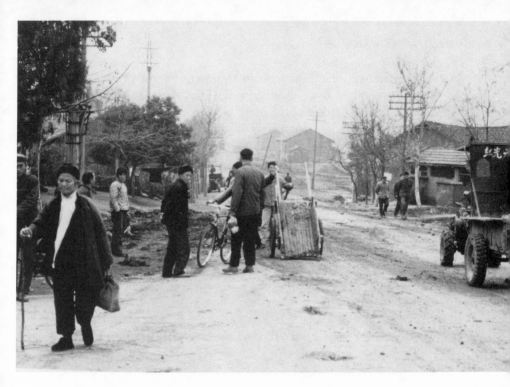

Scene from a commune in the Second Attached Hospital referral area.

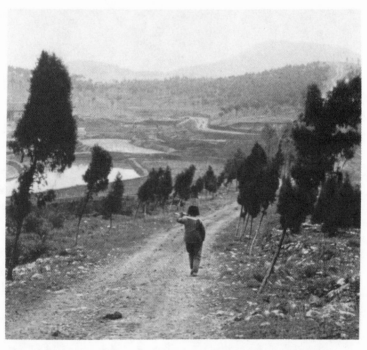

Scene from a commune in the Second Attached Hospital referral area.

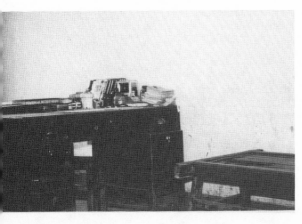

A barefoot doctor's office in a rural production brigade. Attached to the office is a small dispensary stocked primarily with traditional medicines.

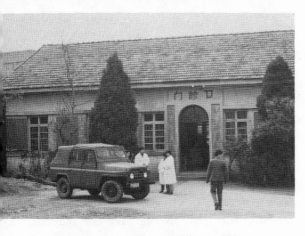

A commune hospital. Barefoot doctors refer patients to outpatient clinics for medical, surgical, and dental care.

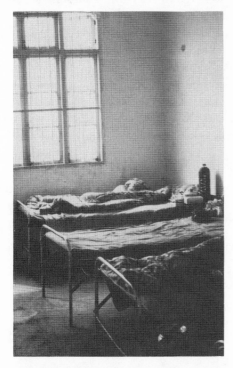

A ward in a commune hospital for patients requiring admission.

7

The Institution and the Patients: Who's in Charge?

ADMISSION TO THE INFECTIOUS DISEASE WARD

All patients come first to the outpatient department of the SAH, which sees a thousand patients each day. The outpatient department, located near the entrance to the hospital, along East Lake Road, is in a two-story rectangular building whose yellow paint has mostly faded away. Inside, the medical departments are located off dark hallways, which are lined with benches for waiting patients. The emergency department, a smaller but considerably more cheerful setting, is located on the right-hand side of the building. A small circular drive in front is crowded with vehicles, vendors, and patients, especially in the early morning, when they line up for their registration numbers. Nonemergency patients are free to select the traditional Chinese medicine department or the Western medicine department. The registration fee for each is .05 yuan. All the patients we interviewed on the infectious disease ward said that those who come to the outpatient departments are well aware of the divisions within Western style medicine; that is, someone with an eye problem will be referred to an eye doctor, someone with a stomach problem to a gastroenterologist.

Patients cannot select a particular physician but are examined by one of the hospital doctors assigned to outpatient department duty. After the examination, the physician makes his or her recommendations. Some patients are sent away with no diagnosis; others are given a prescription for medicine; some are told to rest at home. In the last case, the physician writes the diagnosis in the patient's medical record book (*bingqing zhengmingshu*),[1] which the patient then takes to his or her work unit doctor, who will give

1. The patients keep these medical histories, which record illness, date, opinion, and diagnosis.

permission to be absent from work. For a patient difficult to diagnose, the physician may recommend remaining several days in the outpatient infirmary for more tests. If the illness requires admission to the hospital, the physician alone decides to which department the patient should be admitted and, after checking to make sure there is an available bed, telephones to the ward to request an admission. A nurse from the ward is sent over to escort the patient, first to the hospital accounting department and then to the ward itself. The patient makes a deposit of fifteen yuan to cover the cost of meals for about a month.[2] The head nurse, or someone in her place if she is busy, gives the patient a brief orientation to the ward and its rules.[3] Then a bed, pajamas, and other basic necessities are assigned, and the patient settles into his or her surroundings. This process is abbreviated if the patient is critically ill.

ON THE WARD: PATIENTS AND STAFF

For the majority of patients, who are classified as mildly ill, the ward resembles a convalescent care facility more than a hospital inpatient ward. Medical delegations visiting other types of wards in China have noted the same phenomenon. The mildly ill patients are all ambulatory, and most of them are dressed in street clothes, even under their quilts. They are responsible for their own toilet. They stand at their ward room doors at mealtime to receive their food from the health aides. They wash out their own plates and cups. Many also wash their own clothes and sweep out their ward room floors. During the day, they stroll about in the adjacent courtyard, talk to fellow ward patients, knit, or read. One foreign visitor to our ward remarked with a puzzled tone, "It's so quiet. Where is all the hustle and bustle?" A Western physician visiting another hospital in China noted, "I am struck by the number of not so ill patients there . . . and the longer stay of kids. Many seemed to not need hospitalization." (Committee on Scholarly Communication with the People's Republic of China, 1973, 154–55). People on our ward are not rushed anywhere. Once admitted, they remain an average of thirty days.[4]

2. See Chap. 6, n. 16 for the cost of typical meals.
3. For example, patients are not allowed behind the nursing station and cannot look at their charts, and quiet must be maintained on the ward. Other regulations are explained, including the procedure for ordering food, the visiting hours (only on Sunday on our ward), use of the courtyard, and the rotation of TV watching privileges among the eight ward rooms.
4. This average length of stay contrasts with nineteen days for all patients admitted to the SAH in 1979. The greater length of stay on the infectious disease ward can be attributed to government regulations regarding hospitalization for infectious diseases, particularly hepatitis.

For the seriously and critically ill patients, the ward serves a more conventional function. These patients receive careful nursing attention, in fact more nursing attention than those in many other parts of the hospital. Because the patients are considered contagious, except in the most critical cases relatives are not allowed to care for the patients as they do on other wards. The nurses complain a little about this, but they also admit their jobs are simpler when they do not have to deal with family members.

Does the sick person in China adopt the traditional passive role of obediently accepting treatment? Or does the patient (still under the influence of Cultural Revolution rhetoric) enter into an egalitarian or even challenging relationship with the medical staff? As our observations of the *danwei* had led us to expect, politics was less important than traditional social norms. The following case introduces the nature of the practitioner-client relationship.

One morning, we went to see a nineteen-year-old girl with epidemic hemorrhagic fever. She was in the fever phase, and her face was flushed. She was also extremely embarrassed to have the physicians examine her. She moaned and cried constantly, as if slightly delirious. The head nurse, who was usually exceedingly gentle with patients, was curt. When we asked if she was in pain, the head nurse said no quite sternly. The girl was more upset than actually in pain. With all the physicians and nurses standing around her bed, the nurse said, "She is not a good patient." A physician explained, within easy hearing of the patient, "Not all patients do as they're told [*tinghua*]."

This girl was the youngest of five children, the baby of her family. Her mother was there taking care of her. When we asked the head nurse why the mother was there, she explained that patients could have relatives come onto the ward if they were critically ill or if the nurses refused to care for them. This girl belonged to the second category. The mother sat quietly beside the girl's bed. Her daughter had been moaning about the smell of the disinfectant used to mop the floors (admittedly a pungent odor), and the mother held a handkerchief over the girl's nose.

Tinghua was used often to describe desired patient behavior; it translates as "do as you are told," "be obedient," literally, "listen to what is said." Most commonly, *tinghua* is used to describe children who obey their parents. Likewise, parents also lament the decline in the number of children who still *tinghua*.

Clearly, the ward staff places heavy emphasis on patient compliance and cooperation. In another case, a young male hepatitis patient was criticized in much the same way as the girl described above. The nurses discussed his refusal to cooperate (*ta bu hezuo*) as a main factor in his imminent demise. In fits of delirium, he pulled out his IV and refused to take his medicines. The nurses were angry with him. One said, "He has no hope. He might have if only he would cooperate."[5] The ward staff did, however, excuse behavior that reflected genuine loss of control due to illness. For example, we were told that the physician in charge and the head nurse would surely have criticized the young girl with epidemic hemorrhagic fever very directly had she not been slightly confused. In general, however, physicians and nurses expect patients to accept without question and quietly the treatment they are given. They were amused to note our surprise at the restraint Chinese women show during labor, and at the calm cooperation of patients subjected to uncomfortable sigmoidoscope procedures.

Not surprisingly, this authority relationship between practitioner and client is accompanied by the assumption that the less the patient knows, the better. If one believes that a patient gets better faster by behaving well, then the recovery will proceed even more quickly if the patient is not "upset" by concerns relating to the illness. If a physician needs to discuss a patient's case, it is the relatives who are consulted, not the patient.

Another example of physicians protecting their patients from worrisome news occurred in a different setting. An eighty-year-old college professor suffered what appeared to be a very mild stroke at a dinner party. Both the campus physician and the professor's daughter, a physician at a nearby hospital, were called. Despite their suspicions, they assured the professor that she was overtired and suffering from a cold (*ganmao*). Confused about being confined to bed rest for a week and then to her home for several months, the woman pressed for an explanation. The physicians persisted in their original diagnosis, saying they did not want to worry her further.

In sum, medical personnel seem to believe that patients should know as little as possible about diagnosis, medication, and treatment. When we first arrived on the ward, we noted that the physicians wrote in English in the patient charts and concluded that they did this to facilitate our work. Later one of our colleagues explained, "We write in English so patients don't know what they are getting. Even some outpatient prescriptions are written in this way."[6] As we saw earlier, this attitude extends also to the resolution of medical errors. Unless circumstances force them to, physicians rarely in-

5. Medically, it was not at all certain that if the patient had "behaved" he would have improved.
6. Physicians on other wards also wrote medication orders in patient charts in English.

form a patient of a medical mistake. Rather, after telling the leaders, it falls under the unit's jurisdiction. The physician may hear from an unhappy patient—or, more commonly, the patient's relatives—but it is the institution that will deal with the problems.

THE PATIENT AS A CONSUMER

There is little question that the patients on our ward were rewarded for passive, dependent behavior, but this observation does not imply that they were completely at the mercy of the ward staff. As we have already seen, Chinese patients often take an active role in their health care paths outside the ward, and it would be surprising to observe complete abdication of authority to the ward staff. Notions about patient behavior in the United States can throw some light on the relationship of patient to staff.

Talcott Parsons was the first to define what it means to be sick, in a sociological sense. He wrote that the "sick role" has four basic behaviorial assumptions: (1) exemption from normal social role responsibilities, in accordance with the nature and severity of the illness; (2) the institutionalized expectation that the sick person cannot be expected to get well by an act of will—rather, the person is in a condition that must be taken care of; (3) the definition of the state of being ill as undesirable, with its obligation to want to get well; and (4) the obligation—again in proportion to the severity of the condition—to seek technically competent help and to cooperate with the person selected in the process of trying to get well (Parsons 1951, 314; summarized in Twaddle 1969, 5). Regarding patient behavior on the ward, what is relevant is the notion that the patient is not responsible for being ill but is responsible for seeking help and cooperating with that help in order to get well. The patient expectations that we observed were consistent with, and in some cases extreme examples of, the sick role defined by Parsons.

Until recently, the relationship between patient and practitioner has been defined as inherently asymmetrical. The patient is dependent on the physician's technical knowledge, and the "competence gap" between doctor and patient is said to "justify both the professional's assumption of authority, and the client's trust, confidence and . . . obedience" (Haug and Lavin 1981, 213). Because of the "competence gap," the consumer of medical services is said to delegate his or her freedom of choice to the physician and to "professional standards" to define what service is actually needed (Stevens 1974, 37).

The sick role and the model of professional power over clients have been challenged on several fronts. Most relevant to our purposes is the alternative model of the patient as a consumer of medical services. Haug and Lavin (1981) argue that a significant minority of patients have become increasingly capable of evaluating the performance and competence of the physician and other health care providers. As a result of this challenge, some physicians have modified their own behavior to the extent that the interaction has changed. Haug and Lavin assert that for some interactions, a bargaining model is more appropriate than a dominance model. Physicians bring to the interaction their knowledge, experience, access to services and medications, and a tradition of authority. Patients bring "their knowledge, experience, their threat to take their business elsewhere, and their institutionalized right to 'informed consent' before invasive procedures are instituted" (Haug and Lavin 1981, 214).[7] The traditional authority relationship is still common, but it is now seen to depend on such variables as age, education, experience, and the socialization of the actors involved.

The bargaining perspective offers important insights into any interaction between groups or individuals. Earlier, we have seen the unit members as actors who rely on certain strategies in dealing with units and unit leaders, but who are also constrained by a dearth of exit options. We shall now analyze client strengths in terms of the kind of experience and knowledge that patients believe they bring to the interaction, the ways in which problems are resolved through voice, and exit options, including the option of alternative care.

PATIENT'S RESOURCES: INFORMATION, VOICE, AND EXIT

Information is the key factor in creating intelligent consumers. One way for the patient to cope with the basically asymmetrical physician—patient relationship is to increase his or her ability to make informed decisions *with* the physician (Stevens 1974, 39). Our observations indicate that the overwhelming tendency of Chinese physicians is to provide the patient with the minimum amount of information needed to understand his or her illness. On the other hand, patients on the infectious disease ward exhibited a rather impressive amount of information about and understanding of their disease processes. Although patients were forbidden to see their hospital charts, each patient carried a booklet with a summary of the medical history; and each patient, whether uneducated peasant or sophisticated urbanite, could

---

7. See also Parsons (1975), Haug and Sussman (1969), Stimson and Webb (1975), Freidson (1975), and Carleton (1978).

rattle off the events in his or her case, medications, laboratory tests, and indicators of illness. With this accumulated information and the opinions of
friends and relatives, they formed an evaluation of their medical care. Patients seemed surprisingly well versed in Western as well as Chinese traditional modes of therapy, and many referred to their negative perception of
physician performance at other hospitals or lower-level clinics. In addition,
as we saw in chapter 6, at least some of the patients initiated treatment or
referral themselves.

Chinese patients' sense of confidence as they attempt to understand and
evaluate their medical treatment is further bolstered by a national policy that
encourages self-education in all spheres. This policy reflects a long-standing
emphasis on self-reliance, as well as the regime's periodic philosophical difficulties over how to incorporate professionals whom they believe to be inherently elitist into an egalitarian socialist ideal. The self-education policy
has been most visible during the antiprofessional, radically egalitarian periods of modern Chinese politics, most notably in the Great Leap Forward
and the Cultural Revolution. Since the Cultural Revolution, self-education
has continued to be a major means of making up for education lost during
that decade. Everywhere in China, one encounters self-taught English
teachers, technicians, artists, and healers. Each morning on the national television, education classes are offered in English language, in sciences, and in
other fields. In some factories, workers who pass special examinations are allowed time off to attend this TV college. The reinstitution of qualifying examinations for training programs, university entrance, and employment opportunities has produced an abundance of people teaching themselves a
wide variety of subjects. The message is clear: information is available to
those who apply themselves in learning it.

Self-education in medicine may be particularly acceptable because of
the attempts to integrate Chinese traditional and Western medicine. Beginning in the early fifties, traditional practitioners were encouraged to join the
Western institutions of medicine and to share their knowledge so that the
wealth of the Chinese heritage could be displayed, examined, and validated
as China's unique contribution to medicine. Particularly during the Cultural
Revolution, medical personnel were encouraged to investigate traditional
herbal remedies and to experiment with new varieties. Barefoot doctors and
local neighborhood paramedics (the antithesis of the professional, Western-
trained researcher) were pictured in short stories and novels as pathfinders
in medical research.[8]

8. See, for example, Yang, *The Making of a Peasant Doctor*.

The phenomenon of self-taught healers and the appeal of less expensive traditional medicines have persisted, especially on the local level and in rural areas. Several of the patients on the infectious disease ward mentioned being treated by neighbors or friends who had taught themselves something about traditional Chinese medicines and therapy. Indeed, this practice appears at all levels. One of the physicians on our ward was also a self-taught expert on traditional medicines. During the Cultural Revolution, some observers questioned the quality of the newly trained barefoot doctors, who were encouraged to teach themselves, as well as the lack of supervision of these paramedics (Hsu 1971). On our ward, when a patient reported having visited a neighbor who was self-taught in some local therapy, the responses from fellow patients and the ward staff were mixed.[9] Still, self-education was more often viewed as harmless or helpful rather than evil, and the persistence of support for self-education represents a positive force encouraging patients to acquire medical information on their own, apart from the medical establishment.

Thus self-education and other sources of information provide the patient with certain resources in an encounter with a physician. This fact does not, of course, tell us whether physicians will respond by negotiating directly with patients about their medical care. In the United States, patient advocates have tried to eliminate the "competence gap" between physician and client by passing protective laws and generating consumer participation movements (Stevens 1974, Haug and Lavin 1981). Patients in China do not seem to be pursuing similar strategies.

The second patient resource is the use of indirect voice in decision making and in conflict resolution. As described above, when problems with a patient arise or an important decision must be made, physicians are unlikely to deal directly with the patient; instead, they contact the patient's relatives.[10] Informed consent in China involves the family and the unit, not the individual. Friends, relatives, and work unit leaders act on the patient's behalf, so that the patient need not deal directly with the medical personnel. In this way, problems are resolved but the patient is not required to violate the sick role norms of passivity and compliance. Although this strategy pro-

9. When a middle school chemistry teacher, a hepatitis patient on our ward, described the history of the large blister on his wrist, brought about by moxibustion (cupping), all the other patients in the ward crowded around to give their opinions. Some said he was foolish to have believed that draining the pus would eliminate his jaundice. Some told of friends they knew who had done the same thing.

10. This behavior reflects the traditional cultural norms of avoiding face-to-face conflict through use of an intermediary. See Solomon (1971) for discussion of the persistence of these norms in China since 1949.

vides the patient with a significant resource in resolving conflict, it also severely limits his or her power to negotiate directly with the physician.

Despite regulations to the contrary, when a patient is critically ill one
relative is allowed on the infectious disease ward. Often the nearest kin
sleeps in the bed next to the patient and helps provide nursing care. On the
other wards in the hospital, this is common practice. Whether they are actually on the ward or not, however, relatives are a force with which the medical staff must contend. For example, when we asked the physicians why
a particular drug was prescribed for hepatitis patients when the doctors
all agreed it had no great effect, one replied, "We must give them something Western, or their relatives will criticize us." Physicians are justifiably
wary of the complaints of relatives, which can cause problems with their
own leaders.

In cases of serious dissatisfaction, the patients and their families can
"raise an opinion" (*tiyi*) with their own unit leader about the treatment received. The leader will investigate, generally by contacting the hospital leadership on an individual basis. If the accusation is very serious, a meeting will
be held at the hospital to discuss the case. Usually the leaders involved will
reach an agreement, and if some wrongdoing on the part of the hospital staff
is revealed, then a cash settlement will be offered. If the patient and family
are still not satisfied, they can appeal to higher authorities, or perhaps write
a letter to the newspaper to focus public attention on the case. In these
cases, the appropriate government agency or the newspaper will investigate
to hear both sides. The story will be printed only after the investigators' superiors have given their approval. We heard that such an incident had
occurred shortly before we arrived. A county hospital patient had an operation and later developed what was diagnosed as a tumor. She was referred
to the provincial hospital obstetrics department, and when a second operation was performed, a gauze dressing was found, apparently forgotten by
the first surgeon. It was necessary to inform the patient of the actual nature
of her "tumor." Her family wrote to the leader of the county hospital. The
patient's unit leader came to investigate personally, looked at the chart, and
discussed with the county hospital leadership the compensation due the patient and penalty due the physician. The final decision had not been made
when we left, but it seemed likely that some financial offer would be made
to the patient and that because the error of the physician was unintentional,
the penalty would not be severe.

We observed two instances in which the patient's work unit leader took
an active role in patient care, just as a family member might have done. One

of these involved a thirty-eight-year-old male cadre in the Huanggang District Department of Industry and Commerce, about sixty kilometers from the SAH, who was suffering from viral hepatitis. When he became ill, he went to his district hospital. There hepatitis was diagnosed, and he was admitted to the hospital's infectious disease ward. After one week, however, his unit leader from the Commerce Department felt he was not improving quickly enough and that the facilities and physicians at the SAH were superior to those of the district hospital. Consequently, the unit leader arranged for the patient's transfer to the SAH, the upward referral hospital for this district. Fourteen days after admission to the infectious disease ward, the patient was moved to surgery to explore the possibility of pancreatic cancer.

The second case, a forty-nine-year old male cadre in administration work in a nearby electric wire factory in Wuchang, was likewise suffering from viral hepatitis. When he became ill, he went to his unit's clinic. After developing signs of jaundice, he was sent to the SAH outpatient department for examination and remained there for several days under observation. The outpatient department physicians prepared to admit him to surgery, believing the problem to be gallstones. At this point his factory manager became actively involved in the referral. This leader argued with the physicians that it was not certain that gallstones were the problem, and that the patient's health could not stand an unnecessary operation. A few days later, tests indicated a diagnosis of hepatitis, and the patient was admitted to the infectious disease ward, where he stayed for thirty-three days.

These two incidents illustrate the extent to which other individuals can become involved in health care services, as well as the potential importance of the unit leader in obtaining quality care. Although two cases cannot provide us with general conclusions, it is worth noting features that they had in common: both patients involved were cadres from relatively large units—in one case, a government unit—and the assistance offered by the unit leaders was clearly of benefit. We do not know whether unit leaders would have involved themselves to the same degree on behalf of ordinary workers or other lower-level personnel in their *danwei*, or whether leaders from smaller or rural areas would have the same influence in such matters.

Patients occasionally take action themselves by violating the norms of patient cooperation. Patients are expected to behave passively, but the ward staff do not always respond aggressively to noncompliance. In several instances, physicians seemed to retreat or give up when patients chose not to cooperate. The young female patient mentioned earlier would not *tinghua*, but the physicians did not actively intervene. The introduction of her mother onto the ward could be interpreted as a way to avoid rather than confront the problem of an unmanageable patient.

The third and final resource available to patients in their interaction with physicians is their ability to exit. Under a market system, exit often serves as a powerful instrument by which consumers can express their opinions and influence providers of goods or services (Hirschman 1970). Exit may be less effective when professionals are offering services to clients (Stevens 1974). In the United States, physicians in private practice are affected more by negative feedback from colleagues, particularly if colleagues fail to refer patients, than by the exit of individual patients. This fact has led scholars to conclude that professionals can circumvent basic market mechanisms, with the result that those who purchase their services are at a disadvantage (Freidson 1970a, Stevens 1974, Gross 1977). Given these limitations, we ask what exit options are available to patients in the (nonmarket) Chinese context and whether these alternatives are significant.

Exit Options within the System

The referral system seems to offer few alternatives or exit options for dissatisfied patients. Patients are manuevering within a highly regulated system, and the majority of both urban and rural patients appear to follow the prescribed referral routes and do not attempt to seek out other options, even when they are not happy with their treatment. Yet a certain minority take a more active role. Some patients do not seem to be constrained by the referral rules; they are able to initiate transfer to other hospitals or to intervene in some way in their health care. Urban patients from large work units have a choice of two or three referral sites. For peasants and others from the countryside, the main constraints on health care alternatives seem to be distance and cost rather than the referral regulations. Finally, until very recently, the requirement that patients obtain a referral slip from their local clinic before going to a higher-level facility has not been strictly enforced in either the city or the countryside.

This range of choices available to patients is further augmented by the government's attempt to integrate two previously competing types of health care. The success of this effort and the emphasis on one mode at the expense of the other have varied over time (Lampton 1977, M. Rosenthal 1981). During the Cultural Revolution, for example, emphasis on the traditional medical system obstructed the development of Western-style medicine, which has since regained dominance.

Despite the claim that traditional and Western medicines have been combined, we observed two fundamental dichotomies. First, the lower levels tend to rely on traditional medicines and therapies more than the higher levels. Second, in medical centers and their affiliated teaching hospitals, a division between the two medical systems persists.[11] This incomplete integration appears to offer additional choices to patients attempting to meet their health care needs within the system. Several of the patients described in chapter 6 took advantage of these alternatives when they perceived management of their illnesses to be inadequate. It is noteworthy, though, that the two systems are often viewed as noncompeting therapies. Most of the patients interviewed on the infectious disease ward believed that traditional and Western therapies offered treatment for different disease processes. Western medicines were said to be most appropriate for acute illness, while traditional medicines worked better for chronic problems.[12] When one failed, there was recourse to the other, and patients did not object to being treated with both therapies simultaneously.

Finally, patients may choose between traditional and Western medicine only before admission to the hospital or after discharge. During the course of treatment on a ward, decisions regarding therapy lie solely with the physician. In our interviews with seventy-six patients, none reported having attempted to intervene actively in the treatment they were receiving while they

11. The first dichotomy is illustrated by observations that patients who attend barefoot doctor clinics or neighborhood health stations receive inexpensive traditional therapy and herbal medications (Hsu 1971). The organization of the tertiary-care facilities in Wuhan illustrates the second dichotomy. The majority of these facilities, including the municipal hospitals and teaching hospitals attached to Hubei Provincial Medical College, are what the Chinese call Western-style hospitals. All departments but one are organized like hospitals in the West, with personnel trained in the practice of Western medicine; the one remaining department combines both therapies. This division, however, is somewhat misleading. At the SAH, patients on all wards often receive a combination of traditional and Western medications, and consultations occur between the Western-style wards and the combined ward. Likewise, on the combined ward, physicians with knowledge of Western therapies work beside those trained in traditional medicine. Thus, there has been a trend toward making use of the traditional medicine throughout the hospitals, but the overall thrust and training are toward Western medicine.

The Chinese Traditional Medicine College and its attached hospital provide an alternative for patients purchasing medical services within the established medical system. The hospital, however, incorporates important Western-style therapies, most of its departments are organized in Western style, and many of its staff are trained in both Western and traditional medicine. Here, however, the major emphasis in practice and research is on traditional medicine.

12. One patient quoted a traditional saying to substantiate his opinion that Western medicine should be applied first, to cure superficial symptoms, and Chinese traditional medicine afterward, to deal with the basic nature of illness: "*Xian zhi biao, hou zhi ben*" ("First cure surface, then cure base").

were on our ward. On the contrary, one patient who was taking Western medication for gallbladder problems said that he would like to be seen by a traditional medicine physician as well, but because the infectious disease ward was part of internal medicine (Western medicine), he thought such a request would be "impolite."

Exit Options outside the System

There are three different types of doctors who practice outside the state system of medical care: the licensed traditional Chinese medicine doctor, who has chosen not to join the state medical establishment but rather to practice independently; the so-called native doctor (*tu yisheng*), who is not licensed by the government but practices locally with little government interference; and the witch doctor (*wu yisheng*), who practices illegally.

Because all medical school graduates in China practice medicine within the state system, there are no licensing examinations or certification procedures. The only physicians subject to licensing are older, traditional practitioners who have decided to continue their old-style practice. Many were trained at a medical school or under an apprenticeship to a master practitioner for five or six years. Their decision to be independent of the system may be related to a desire to keep their prescriptions secret or to avoid the pressure of learning all aspects of medicine, or they may have preferred not to be part of a state apparatus. Some have set up their practice in an office or clinic; some travel to where the clients congregate. One of these physicians often came to the grounds directly in front of the SAH outpatient department. There he laid out a blanket, set down his license, which stated that he was a doctor licensed by the government, and described the diseases he was certified to treat. These physicians appear to be quite popular. We heard several tales of miraculous cures by traditional practitioners who could rejoin broken bones or help diabetes faster than Western physicians.

The most important issue, of course, is not whether these practitioners are effective, but whether they are regarded as a real choice or alternative to the established system. Our limited inquiries indicate that for some people with some diseases, the traditional practitioners offer a viable exit from the state system. For many diseases, particularly acute syndromes, however, patients probably have little choice but to enter the established medical institutions.

Native doctors, who are usually peasants, are more limited in their repertoire and generally do not make their living practicing medicine. For friends and neighbors or for people who have a correct introduction, they prescribe herbal remedies passed on through parents and grandparents. Several people stressed that these doctors are under no obligation to see patients and in fact refuse to treat some people. The method of payment also indicates the different nature of the relationship. After treatment, patients generally present gifts rather than money. Treatment by native doctors is thus more of a favor to friends than a client-practitioner relationship. According to the infectious disease physicians, the government does not concern itself with either licensing or regulating these doctors, apparently considering them fairly harmless.

Several patients on the ward, with hepatitis, had experience with native doctors: One, a forty-four-year-old cadre working in administration in an electronics factory, first had hepatitis in 1965. After an unsuccessful seven-month stay in the Chinese Traditional Medicine College hospital in Wuhan, he simply went home thinking the doctors could not cure him. Friends at home introduced him to a peasant doctor whose father collected herbs for traditional medicine. He charged no fee. This native doctor made a medicine with tree and grass roots, to be eaten twice daily, then applied a poultice to the patient's wrist to bring up a large blister. After puncturing the blister and draining the yellow fluid, he pronounced the patient cured. Although the patient had little faith in this cure, subsequent laboratory tests showed that he no longer had hepatitis. His second case of hepatitis was diagnosed at the SAH outpatient department, but the cadre was reluctant to be admitted. Only after representatives from the Disease Prevention Station (under the Bureau of Public Health) visited him at home was he persuaded to enter the hospital. He stayed forty days.

The last category practicing outside the state-run medical institutions is the witch doctor, literally translated "evil (or bad) doctor." As the name implies, these practitioners are considered to be charlatans, and they travel around the countryside. We were told that most are women and that they act as though medicine were their profession but have no medical training and sell prescriptions of their own formulation. One physician said that sometimes there are newspaper reports of a patient who has died at the hands of a witch doctor, and the doctor is subsequently arrested by the government. Even when it is known that these doctors are not honest or adequately trained, the government does not become involved unless a patient has been hurt or killed by the treatment. Likewise, the hospital did not seem to have any policy regarding witch doctors but tried on an individual basis to educate patients who had come in contact with them. None of the patients we talked to had visited a witch doctor.

Thus, it appears that the impact of patient exit on the provider of the service is small, and probably much smaller within the state-run institutions than with traditional practitioners outside the system. In the nonmarket Chinese economy, both the salaries of physicians and other medical staff and the referral of patients are fixed. In tertiary-care facilities such as the SAH, beds are rarely empty, and if they are, the physician's income, position, and bargaining power with patients are not adversely affected. Any resulting decrease in the workload is a short-term positive effect.

These observations allow us to add to the general conclusions about exit and voice discussed in chapter 5. In the hospital *danwei* itself, unit leaders do not readily respond to the staff's exercise of voice, because the threat of staff exit is small. Faced with this situation, the unit staff tend to use indirect voice, including group voice and "raising an opinion" to an outside authority, to influence events in the unit. The position of patients is somewhat different. They are brought into the unit for a brief time and appear to have a fair degree of flexibility and mobility within the referral system. Like the unit staff members, they are constrained in the use of voice, but for patients the major constraints are the dictates of the sick role and the tendency of health care providers to supply as little information as possible in direct negotiation. Furthermore, we saw no evidence that increased information placed the patients in a more advantageous position. Patients may make use of the exit option when they are dissatisfied, but the threat of exit does not appear to improve the patient's position vis-à-vis the health care provider, either because exit alternatives may not be appropriate to the illness or because patient exit has little effect on the physician. Instead, strategies similar to those employed by unit staff—the use of indirect voice and the intervention of outsiders—seem to have the greatest impact on the practitioners and the delivery of care.

DISCHARGE

When the patient has recovered sufficiently to warrant discharge, the physician writes in the chart, "Patient should leave tomorrow."[13] The nurses send the chart to the pharmacy for calculation of the cost of medicine, then to the accountant for calculation of the other items on the bill, such as room, heat, procedures, and laboratory tests. Food is totaled separately and the patient is either charged or refunded the difference, based on the initial

13. For many of the infectious diseases, the Ministry of Health has set regulations for patient discharge.

deposit. Bills of patients with complete medical insurance coverage are sent to their work unit to pay. Peasants, temporary workers, workers in small collectively owned enterprises, and dependents with only partial medical coverage must pay the bill in full before they leave the hospital. They will then submit the receipt to their work units or commune administrators for the reimbursement to which they are entitled.

Patients, who sometimes must pay large amounts, borrow money from relatives, their work unit, or commune funds and then slowly repay the loan. One scholar conducting interviews of immigrants in Hong Kong cites unpaid hospital bills as a major source of peasant debt.[14] The state hospital budget includes an allowance for patients who are unable to pay their hospital bills (fifty yuan per bed per year). We also heard stories of sympathetic doctors who helped peasants who could not pay their bills to escape out the back door of the hospital.

DEATH AND AUTOPSY

Not all patients, of course, leave the ward alive. Of the eighty-four patients on the infectious disease ward during our study, six percent died. The death rate for the entire hospital in 1979 was reported at 3.7 percent. After patients have died, their bodies are taken to a morgue to await removal by relatives. Cremation is recommended by the regime, but burial still occurs commonly in the countryside.

Traditional attitudes also prevail in the matter of autopsy. It is difficult to convince the relatives of a patient to give up the body for examination. One physician told us, "During the Cultural Revolution autopsies were particularly rare. We didn't want to make waves, so no one asked for them. Even now, the *laobaixing* [common folk] don't like them. They want the whole corpse returned." When physicians feel an autopsy is especially important for understanding the nature of a disease or the cause of death, they use a variety of approaches to convince relatives to allow one.

Generally, the hospital offers some form of financial compensation for an autopsy and also provides for the cost of cremation.[15] The amount of compensation seems to vary depending upon the willingness of the relatives and their financial needs. One urban family was offered a set fee of 100 yuan. Another family, from the countryside, was initially unwilling to allow

14. Jean C. Oi (personal communication).
15. The cost of cremation is generally paid by the patient's work unit. Perhaps this benefit is offered by the hospital as an extra incentive for those without *danwei* death benefits.

autopsy, and the hospital offered to reimburse them for their relative's entire hospital bill of 380 yuan. This situation was not resolved before we left China, but because the patient's husband was fearful of his mother-in-law's reaction, the offer was probably turned down. We were told that for cases considered quite important, the hospital will also go to the leaders of the relative's unit(s) to gain their assistance in persuading the relatives. Occasionally these tactics produce an undesired effect. In one case we were told about, the parents of a girl who had died of hepatitis offered her body to the hospital in exchange for 400 yuan and a job for the girl's mother. When the hospital leaders refused this proposal, the parents hung a large poster (*dazibao*), complete with cartoon, at the hospital entrance saying that the physician taking care of their daughter had killed her by giving an incorrect injection.[16] After a visit from the head of the hospital, the parents retracted their claims and the matter was dropped.

SUMMARY

For patients who have been admitted to a hospital ward, the relationship with hospital personnel, and especially with physicians, is asymmetrical. Patients are required to conform to the sick role and to cooperate with medical decisions made by physicians. The prevailing belief is that the less the patient knows, the better. Relatives are contacted for medical consultations and informed consent.

Patients have resources for exercising control over their situation. Noncompliance may be one method of influencing care, because sanctions are not severe. Relying on information accumulated from their own experiences and friends and relatives, patients may decide that the care they are receiving is inadequate and go elsewhere for help. Exiting may improve their immediate situation, but it seems to have little impact on the basic hierarchical practitioner-client relationship; in this nonmarket setting where demand exceeds supply, physicians are affected little. The most powerful resource patients have is the assistance of friends, relatives, and leaders who act on their behalf. Physicians on our ward seemed to react strongly to criticism by relatives, and they admitted that relatives affected their prescribing habits. Finally, the patients' work unit leaders can serve not only as potential advocates but also as final arbitrators for disputes between patients and those who provide medical care.

16. Big character posters were common protest devices during the Cultural Revolution.

8

Practicing Medicine

Just as a factory *danwei* exists in order to turn out a product, so our unit existed in order to provide and support sophisticated (tertiary) health care. Here we compare this "product," the current practice of medicine in China, with a similar setting in the United States and with earlier reports about Chinese medical care by Western physicians and scientists. Our discussion covers several stages of patient care: history taking and physical examination, diagnostic formulation, and patient management. Medical education and traditional Chinese therapy will also be considered.

THE INITIAL INTERACTION: HISTORY AND PHYSICAL EXAMINATION

The history and physical examination represent the point of initial communication between the physician and the patient. In the private practice of medicine in the United States, patients who require hospitalization generally receive both outpatient and inpatient care from the same physician. In an institutional setting, however (such as at North Carolina Memorial Hospital), care is transferred from the examining physician in the emergency room or the outpatient clinic to the ward physician. The latter type of practice is the norm in China, where outpatient department doctors are generally on long-term (perhaps permanent) assignments.

At the Second Attached Hospital, the initial examination, diagnosis, and decision for admission are made in the outpatient department, followed by a telephone call to the ward physician responsible for treatment of a specific disease (such as hepatitis). Occasionally, however, patients simply come to the ward door to be admitted. In either case, patients are accompanied by a nurse. As in Western hospitals, patients are assigned a hospital bed and offered instructions by the nurses before a second history and physical examination are undertaken by the ward physician.

In Chinese hospitals, privacy is not a priority (Reynolds 1980). On our ward the beds were close together and generally not separated by curtains. Patients in adjacent beds made no effort to hide their interest in the problems of new admissions, and the physicians did not discourage their curiosity. Most physical examinations were conducted with shared equipment (stethoscope, otoscope), which was kept in a closed cabinet along with a basin of formaldehyde in an attempt to promote sterilization. A few physicians had their own instruments. Privacy during the physical examination itself was less of an issue than during conversation because patients wore several layers of clothing, which hid their anatomy. This "clothed" approach to the physical examination sometimes interfered with thoroughness.

Privacy is even further limited by the presence of relatives and friends visiting the ward. Visitors spent most of their days in the patients' rooms or outside the rooms in the locked courtyard. When the physicians did their work on the wards, visitors would literally hang in through the windows to gain added information. The presence of this audience did not seem to bother the physicians.

At first we perceived this behavior as an egalitarian holdover from the Cultural Revolution. Eventually, however, we concluded that curiosity is simply a deeply ingrained Chinese trait. Our own experience, both during shopping trips to Wuhan and in the hospital, and the experiences of other visitors to China tend to confirm this view. On one occasion we were invited to watch a surgical procedure performed with acupuncture anesthesia, and our translator, who had never witnessed surgery, decided to join us. We stood on a raised platform in the operating room several yards from the patient. Our translator had poor vision and was continually craning her neck to get a better look. While we two foreigners talked to each other, our translator left the platform and leaned over between the surgeon and his assistant in order to get a better look at the incision. She was reprimanded by the surgeons and sent back to the platform. This episode emphasizes how unself-conscious she was about crowding into almost any situation to get a better look at something. The Chinese call this "having a look" (*kanyikan*).

In summary, the history and physical examination are similar to those in the United States except that they tend to be briefer and less private. (In some wards, such as obstetrics and gynecology, examination rooms are available.) The physician's evaluations are then recorded in open-faced charts kept at the nursing station. Records of previous visits and the discharge diagnosis are carefully stored according to a numbering system. These old records, which are very important to medical care, can be retrieved with remarkable accuracy.[1] Although they are not available immediately after the patient's admission, this is not a major problem in China, because patients also carry a detailed medical record book.

DIAGNOSTIC FORMULATION

After the history and physical examination, the physician must come to a decision regarding diagnostic possibilities, the gravity of the illness, and treatment. The list of diagnostic possibilities generated (the differential diagnosis) is used to define essential blood and radiographic tests that can be used to support one diagnosis and, equally important, exclude all others.

It is in its use of laboratory procedures that medicine in China differs most dramatically from that in the West. Like hospitals in most other developing countries, the Second Attached Hospital was quite limited in material resources. All its laboratories were located in rather cramped quarters on the third floor. There was almost no automation. All hematology and clinical chemistry work was done by hand. The microbiology laboratory was adequately stocked with media, but bench space was limited and the facilities were unsophisticated. The instruments that we saw in use (simple spectrophotometers and electrophoresis apparatus, and microscopes) were of Chinese manufacture, so we were not familiar with their quality. The laboratories we visited were busy performing essential tests.

The radiology and nuclear medicine departments were much better equipped than the clinical laboratories. It was clear that both departments had recently been allowed to make major purchases. Radiology had imported several pieces of sophisticated Japanese equipment, and the facilities permitted routine plain films and fluoroscopic contrast procedures (such as barium enemas). There was also equipment to perform and record angiography (blood vessel studies). However, the X-ray film itself and several of the X rays we examined seemed of very poor quality.

The nuclear medicine facility had isotopes and detection equipment ad-

1. An earlier report (Reynolds 1980) questioned whether any patient records were maintained in China. We were able to review records of 134 patients with epidemic hemorrhagic fever admitted to Hubei Provincial Medical College in the years 1970–1980 (Cohen et al. 1981). The infectious disease ward records listed all patients admitted with this disorder and identified patient charts by number. Those were then retrieved from a separate building.

equate for most routine scans. We were unable to ascertain how the isotopes were obtained or disposed of. Several canisters labeled as containing radioactive material were sitting on the ground outside the doors of the facility. Neither the radiology nor nuclear medicine department seemed particularly busy. Some of the advanced equipment we saw may have been purchased more in response to the drive toward modernization than for practical purposes. Some Chinese administrators with whom we talked equated equipment per se with modernization; they were more interested in obtaining these visible markers of high technology than the information necessary for their application. Other Westerners working in China have made similar observations (William A. Fischer, personal communication). More important, the facilities were not busy because physicians in China do not routinely depend on laboratory evaluation for diagnosis or management.

In a Western medical setting, laboratory tests are ordered en masse to exclude each possible disease, and a diagnosis is obtained by the process of elimination. This approach to medicine has been fostered by technological advances, easy access to reliable, quick testing; financial reward for those who perform the tests; and a defensive strategy that takes into consideration the litigious attitude of patients in the United States. Dependence on laboratory testing for diagnosis is phenomenally expensive (Lyle 1979) and is used more frequently by fee-for-service physicians than by those on salary (Able-Smith 1969). Chinese physicians, on the other hand, are comfortable with diagnosis by inclusion. A presumptive diagnosis is entertained based on limited data. A treatment regimen is chosen and diagnosis is confirmed or rejected on the basis of the patient's response. Knaus (1981) has observed the same approach among Soviet physicians.

For a Western physician playing an active role in the care of patients in China, diagnosis by inclusion can be harrowing, as our experience with the two following cases shows.

On 18 November 1979, a thirty-year-old male was transferred to the Second Attached Hospital with a febrile illness. His disease had begun with the acute onset of chills and headache, and a temperature of 41°C was recorded. He was evaluated in a commune clinic and given an intramuscular injection of penicillin. His symptoms persisted and he was admitted to the infectious disease ward three days later. His chest X ray was unremarkable; a complete blood count revealed a white blood count of 26,000/mm³. Urinalysis revealed white blood cells too numerous to count but no bacteria. A prolonged bleeding time was noted. Physical examination showed a young man in moderate discomfort with photophobia, an inflamed pharynx, and mild stiffness of the neck. The Chinese physicians assigned to the patient were confident that he suffered from epidemic hemorrhagic fever, although the urinary abnormalities were limited. In an American hospital such symptoms would lead to an emergency lumbar puncture to exclude bacterial meningitis. Here, however, no further diagnostic studies were undertaken, and only supportive therapy was offered. The patient made an uneventful recovery.

Another patient, a twenty-six-year-old man, was admitted to the infectious disease ward with headache, mild cough, and persistent high fever. He complained of anorexia, mild constipation, and abdominal discomfort. Blood cultures and urine cultures were obtained, and chloramphenicol was prescribed for the presumed diagnosis of typhoid fever. On his second day in the hospital the patient developed more severe abdominal pain, and a diagnosis of colonic perforation was assumed and confirmed at surgery later that evening. Thus, with limited laboratory information, a correct diagnosis was made and a major complication rapidly identified.

The Chinese physicians on the infectious disease ward were undoubtedly familiar with diseases such as epidemic hemorrhagic and typhoid fever; nevertheless, their freedom from dependence on laboratory testing was remarkable. Their approach was formulated on the basis of their experience and available laboratory testing. In theory, this approach would allow some diseases to go undiagnosed and could lead to tragic results. During our brief tenure on the infectious disease ward, however, no such event occurred.

PATIENT MANAGEMENT

In the United States, trials of medication not aimed at a specific diagnosis are usually undertaken in an outpatient setting (as when penicillin is prescribed for fever regardless of the cause). Hospitalization, on the other hand, is directed toward exact diagnosis. This is not the case in China. Again, because of limited resources, there is less emphasis on specific diagnosis and more on speedy intervention, even among inpatients. Furthermore, and perhaps most striking, multidrug therapy is initiated regardless of whether the therapy chosen is of known benefit.

This shotgun approach to therapy has several possible explanations. One is patient expectations. Whereas patients hospitalized in a Western institution expect to undergo a series of tests, the patients we encountered in

China expected to receive "powerful" drugs during their hospitalization: because so little testing was done, there was no other obvious reason for hospitalization. Another is the persistence of physicians' prescribing habits developed during the Cultural Revolution, when these were neither compared
nor controlled and the practice of medicine was, for the most part, secretive.
Physicians who were well trained in Western medicine, and therefore at
greatest risk for criticism, were unlikely to offer advice to a nurse turned
doctor, regardless of how redundant, expensive, or inappropriate the latter's
choice of therapy. The third, and perhaps most important, explanation may
be an effect of mixing traditional and Western medical therapy. Until quite
recently, traditional medical therapy was not subjected to controlled trials
but was employed by historical precedent.

This relaxed attitude in prescribing habits is in striking contrast to the
otherwise curious and critical attitude of Chinese physicians. For example,
they often asked us questions about the application of antimicrobial therapy. In some instances, we found the use of such drugs in China to be inappropriate in terms of choice of drug, amount of dosage, or interval prescribed. Our Chinese colleagues would listen to our comments, review the
subject in Chinese textbooks, and engage in a group discussion of the subject.[2] On most occasions they followed our suggestions. In fact, our recommendations so often agreed with those in Chinese textbooks that we gradually gained clinical credibility on the ward.

No specific therapy is available for the viral illness epidemic hemorrhagic fever (Cohen 1982) or for hepatitis; yet the greatest cost of hospitalization for patients with these diseases is medicines. Overutilization of medications is common in all developing countries (Evans, Hall, and Warford
1981). One example illustrates the wide variety of medications used among
patients we saw. A thirty-year-old male was admitted to the Second Attached
Hospital with a diagnosis of epidemic hemorrhagic fever. During his fifty-
two-day hospitalization he received the following drugs intravenously: hy-
drocortisone, vitamin C, rutin, dicynum, chloramphenicol, furosemide,
mannitol, and cytochrome C. The cost of his hospitalization was 114.17
yuan; medicines accounted for 34 percent of this sum. What is more, their
clinical value was questionable. We observed the same phenomenon in the
treatment of viral hepatitis, in which medication accounted for about 48.5
percent of hospital costs.

2. Textbooks in China are written by expert authors gathered together in a central location by invitation from the national government. Hence, most students and physicians
throughout China use identical reference material. The books we were able to examine were
generally factually correct but did not cite original sources.

Although the Chinese physicians with whom we worked prescribed medications liberally, they were hesitant to perform invasive procedures. In the United States, such hesitation generally relates to difficulty in obtaining informed consent or to fear of malpractice. Neither of these factors seems important in China. The physicians on our ward usually sought permission for procedures from relatives rather than from the patients themselves, and in most cases had no difficulty obtaining it. Malpractice did not seem to be a consideration. Rather, the physicians were reluctant to force a procedure on unwilling patients even if it might clearly be to their benefit.

Several physicians seemed to have had limited experience with what in the West would be considered basic procedures. We got the impression that many of these skills atrophied during the Cultural Revolution. For example, one patient on the ward, a fifty-eight-year-old male with epidemic hemorrhagic fever, developed major gastrointestinal bleeding. Blood count and stool examination reflected blood loss that was not easily monitored or affected by several traditional medications directed at improving coagulation. All the physicians agreed that a nasogastric tube for drainage was appropriate but felt that the patient would not cooperate with its placement. After a lengthy discussion, one of the Chinese physicians halfheartedly attempted to insert the tube and failed. One of us instructed that the patient be restrained, and the nasogastric tube was inserted without difficulty. The patient's gastrointestinal bleeding resolved with nasogastric lavage, and he recovered uneventfully.

In contrast, some diagnostic procedures that are done with difficulty and hesitation in the United States are performed superbly in the People's Republic of China. For example, one morning each week, patients gathered at the outpatient department for diagnostic evaluation of schistosomiasis. The patients would lie stoically on a narrow examining table while rectal biopsy by sigmoidoscopy was performed. The procedure was handled adeptly by the physician we observed, and the biopsy specimen was interpreted immediately in a light microscope. In the United States, this kind of evaluation would require prior laboratory evaluation to exclude any possibility of bleeding (an extremely rare event), informed consent, processing of the specimen by multiple laboratories, and a delay before diagnosis. Clearly, physicians in China and the United States develop different mechanical skills based on the kind of patients they treat, the status of the patient within the system, and patients' perceived rights.

In general, the Chinese ward physicians operated much like U.S. doctors in private practice with small patient loads. After morning rounds, they dispersed to their individual rooms and patients. Although informal discussions of patient-related problems occurred continually in the chart room, formal group rounds (under the supervision of the chief of infectious disease) were held only once or twice a week. When unusual problems developed, senior-level physicians might be asked to make major medical decisions. For example, a thirty-five-year-old Chinese female with epidemic hemorrhagic fever developed severe swelling around the neck, and eventually it became clear that the swelling would interfere with her breathing. A tracheostomy was not feasible because of the bleeding associated with her disorder. The anesthesiology department was asked to insert a noncollapsible tube down the patient's throat and into her lungs, but refused. Debate continued for several hours, until the middle of the night, when the vice-director of the hospital was asked to visit the ward and make a final decision.[3]

The approach in this case illustrates several points. First, it is likely that the leadership status of the vice-director made him an appropriate person to settle a medical debate. Furthermore, he had recognized experience in treating epidemic hemorrhagic fever. In some ways, the solution to this disagreement resembled the one described in chapter 4, in which a physician of lower status was hesitant to offer a correct diagnosis to a physician of higher status.

In the United States, it is rare for physicians to come forth and offer public or private criticism of their colleagues (Freidson 1975). Under these circumstances, it is the patients who suffer. Furthermore, the reluctance of physicians in the United States to police their own ranks has helped to foster the present malpractice dilemma. In the *danwei*, a political figure might have the ability and the legitimacy to intervene in medical practice.

MEDICAL EDUCATION

Undergraduate medical education in China, both during and since the Cultural Revolution, has been described in detail elsewhere (Sidel and Sidel 1973, 1982; Dimond 1971; Cheng et al. 1975; Wen and Hays 1975; Shipp 1982).

---

3. See Cohen et al. (1981) for a more detailed description. This case also illustrates a hazard for a Western physician in China. Having been involved with the care of this patient, we had strong feelings about the appropriate management and a sense of responsibility for the unfortunate outcome. It would have been difficult for a young, foreign physician inexperienced with epidemic hemorrhagic fever to influence the vice-director of the hospital. In our case, public disagreement would have had an adverse effect on the delicate relationships that were forming. Cultural differences, limited diagnostic facilities, lack of experience with endemic diseases, and the *danwei* system can be expected to have a dramatic impact on Western physicians involved in biomedical exchanges.

Postgraduate training in China is similar to that in the United States, but perhaps longer. Formal residence or specialty training is more or less an apprenticeship, with candidates chosen on the basis of interest and accomplishments in accordance with *danwei* and governmental needs (Sidel and Sidel 1982).

As for continued medical education, most of the physicians we met had adequate time for study and were uniformly enthusiastic about acquiring new information. Every member of the ward staff had a plan for further specialty training, either abroad or at a Chinese facility that would afford some unique experience. Physicians consulted existing resources daily. The medical library contained all major Western journals as well as Japanese, Soviet, and Chinese periodicals. However, all foreign materials from the period of the Cultural Revolution were missing, as were any articles pertaining to medicine in China.[4] The libraries we visited had few up-to-date Western textbooks.

Perhaps even more impressive was the number of journals the Chinese physicians read or received in the mail. From an informal survey of physicians studying English we learned that most read three to five foreign journals each month (in their own specialty) and subscribed to two or more Chinese periodicals. Chinese journals abstracting or summarizing English articles have also become available.[5]

Second, and equally important, was the commitment on the part of physicians in the institutions in Wuhan to formal educational experiences. Each physician was allotted one free afternoon per week for educational purposes. Many used this time to attend a local lecture or one at an institution in another part of the city. Hospital lectures were announced by posters, and institutions in the city communicated with each other about them by mail or telephone. Enthusiasm was so great that tickets were required for admission. We gave several formal lectures ourselves. An enormous room inside the medical college was always filled to capacity, mostly with visitors from other institutions who had traveled several hours to attend.[6] The audience was invariably friendly, and eager to offer questions and comments.

4. During our research we attempted to review several articles about China by Western physicians (such as Dimond 1971, Sidel and Sidel 1973). These benign, generally flattering articles were uniformly absent from bound journals. Presumably they had been removed when the journals entered China. We have no idea why.
5. English-language articles were in such great demand that Chinese journals offered an honorarium for free-lance translation.
6. Because so much travel time was involved for those attending lectures, we and others were asked to speak for a minimum of two hours. In our case, translation was also required, so the lectures often lasted three to four hours. Our Chinese audience, however, remained remarkably alert.

Despite these positive elements, major problems afflict continuing medical education in China. In both clinical and basic research, there is extremely poor communication between investigators on a national level. Most work is published in uncirculated institutional journals, or as the minutes of sometimes obscure meetings. Furthermore, some of even the most routine documents are considered internal documents (*neibu*). As such, they are "state secrets" and not accessible to foreign investigators.[7]

Having documented the availability of current information, we were curious as to whether physicians were able or willing to change their prescribing habits. We saw no evidence of interference in this regard from administrators, leaders, or other physicians. As mentioned earlier, if our own suggestions could be substantiated by a reputable Chinese authority, they were adopted without delay. We also observed several uses of Western therapy that had been described only the year before our visit. In general, Chinese physicians seemed quite flexible in their practice of medicine.

TRADITIONAL MEDICINE

The inclusion of traditional and herbal medicine in routine practice has been a continual source of fascination and speculation for Western observers (Horn 1969, Sidel and Sidel 1973, Kleinman 1975, Lee 1981, Lasagna 1975, Quinn 1972, Lampton 1977). Practically speaking, in 1949 there were simply not enough Western-trained physicians to take over the functions performed by traditional practitioners. Furthermore, the Chinese have great faith in traditional medical therapy, which according to at least one Western scholar (Crozier 1968) serves as a focal point of Chinese national pride. Regardless of its effectiveness, traditional medical therapy is both more readily available and cheaper than Western procedures and pharmaceutical agents.

The main problem with Chinese traditional therapies is that they have rarely been standardized or subjected to the scrutiny of controlled trials required for the application of Western therapy. Furthermore, attempts to apply certain traditional procedures in the United States (such as acupuncture for anesthesia or the relief of chronic pain) have been generally unsuccessful (Moore and Berk 1976).

---

7. In our review of epidemic hemorrhagic fever we learned of a national conference held in 1978. We were unable to obtain the minutes of this meeting despite petitions to both Chinese and U.S. embassy authorities. The idea that medical literature might be a state secret puts visiting scientists in the uncomfortable position of having their research possibly considered "spying."

At the Second Attached Hospital, patients were admitted by request to the combined Western and traditional Chinese medicine ward unless they were acutely ill or beds were not available. Most of the physicians on this ward were trained primarily in Chinese traditional practices, and two Western-style physicians were also assigned. We witnessed special classes to teach traditional doctors more Western medicine. On several occasions, patients with infectious diseases (such as epidemic hemorrhagic fever or hepatitis) were transferred from the traditional medicine ward to the infectious disease ward for further care. In careful questioning, we did not detect any critical or condescending attitude among our infectious disease colleagues. One of the physicians on the infectious disease ward had a particular interest in traditional medicine and was self-trained in this area. His advice was frequently sought for our patients. Physicians on our ward also sought official consultations from traditional medical doctors. For example, as described earlier, a patient with hemorrhagic fever and uremia developed persistent uncontrollable hiccups and a course of acupuncture was attempted to relieve the problem.

During our work in China, we avoided extensive involvement with traditional medicine because we had neither the time nor expertise to develop systematic analysis. Traditional practices, however, were ubiquitous, and some impressed even the most skeptical observers.

On several occasions, we were invited to witness acupuncture anesthesia, used in combination with pretreatment barbiturates on patients undergoing stomach, thyroid, and chest surgery. All the patients we witnessed were alert enough to respond to our questions; none were intubated. One such operation involved the removal of a lung from an elderly Chinese male. His ribs were crushed with a large clipping instrument while an assistant used an electric (hot) scalpel to coagulate blood vessels. The room was filled with smoke, and the surgeon was forced to step aside while the patient coughed and cleared his throat.

9

Defining the *Danwei*: Sociological and Medical Significance

Since our return from China in 1980, other physicians and public health educators have written extensively about health care there (Blendon 1981, Sidel and Sidel 1982, Mechanic and Kleinman 1981, Hinman and Parker 1982), and scholars and journalists have commented on the central importance of the *danwei* to urban residents of China (Butterfield 1982; Bernstein 1982; Fraser 1980; Blecher and White 1980; Broyelle, Broyelle, and Tschirhart 1980). We have compared our results and perceptions with theirs. Furthermore, a major study by Whyte and Parish (1983) on urban life in China enabled us to locate our own experiences within the complex reality of urban China. Our study is of one unit, which performed one function, and is subject to the limitations of participant-observation, the methodology best suited to such research. (See appendix 7 for detailed discussion of this methodology and its limitations.) Our findings are necessarily specific to our own *danwei*.

In observing the impact of this urban *danwei* on the organization and delivery of medical care in China, we were initially struck by the regimentation of both the members' and patients' lives—the volume of regulations, the involuntary assignments, the constraints on exit and the crucial role of the leaders. Gradually, however, we perceived varying degrees of flexibility for *danwei* members and clients. In some areas the flexibility was small, as in the degree of individual freedom involved in assignment to the work unit. In others—such as the ability of hospital clients to maneuver within the referral system, or the degree to which *danwei* staff could influence leaders without resorting to confrontation—we found a surprising amount of leeway. The cross-cutting strategies of unit members and clients mitigate the control of individuals by a society that at least one recent author has labeled "intrusive, supervised, molded, centrally planned, totalistic" (Bernstein 1982, 160).

138

DEFINITION OF DANWEI: *A SUMMARY*

Danwei, "work unit," is an administrative term referring to the organization of almost all urban workplaces under the authority of the central government.[1] Originally, the system was established as part of the national plan to restrict migration of rural residents into already crowded cities, to socialize industry and commerce, and to develop a rational system of job allocation and distribution of goods and services. Since then, *danwei* have evolved to serve political and social as well as economic functions. They allow for distribution of jobs, housing, goods, and services to the people. They also serve as the locus of political activity, government surveillance, and communication both from the regime to its citizens and from citizens to their leaders. Gradually, the arena of work unit responsibility has widened to include such diverse areas as personnel assignment, family planning, and the arbitration of disputes. Even during the Cultural Revolution, a social and political movement that attacked many of the conservative elements in socialist China (bureaucracy, elitism, and traditional attitudes), the *danwei* system persisted. Fox Butterfield has called work units "the basic building block of society," observing that "a Chinese is more likely to be asked his *danwei* than his name when he goes someplace new" (1982, 40).

Work units vary enormously in size, function, services, and housing. As Whyte and Parish (1983) point out, the work unit is only one of two systems of urban administration—the other being the urban neighborhood. Indeed, visitors to China have long been aware of the role of the neighborhood committees in the delivery of health care (Sidel and Sidel 1973). For some citizens, work units and neighborhoods are coterminous; for others there is no overlap; for still others there is partial overlap: a couple may live in the work unit of one spouse while the other commutes to a different unit. Unit members we interviewed did not believe that the social meaning of the work unit had moved beyond that of an administrative designation to that of an actual new "village." People's deep ties to their traditional seat of family and kinship had not been severed in a matter of decades.

The work unit system is an *urban* phenomenon. Rural citizens live in households that are part of work teams, in most cases corresponding to natural villages. These are, in turn, organized into brigades (about ten teams)

---

1. Very recently, China has introduced new economic arrangements in urban employment that appear to operate outside the unit system. Licensed vendors or workers engaged in small private enterprises such as restaurants do not belong to units. These are a very small proportion of the urban work force, however.

and communes (about 16,000 members). The work team and the household are the most important administrative levels for planning, distribution of goods and services, and accountability. Comparisons between the rural work team and the urban *danwei* have been made (Oi 1983), but the analogy is complex. Unlike some urban work units, rural work teams always combine territorial and administrative organization. Yet the direct control of the team over its members seems mitigated by both the layered hierarchy of administration and the unique nature of agricultural production. Perhaps the simplest illustration of the difference between urban and rural work organization is the fact that in interviews with ward patients (as well as in their hospital charts), urban patients identified themselves by naming their *danwei*, whereas rural patients named their commune, brigade, and work team.

THE SOCIOLOGICAL SIGNIFICANCE OF THE DANWEI

The 1949 revolution was based on the notion that traditional Chinese culture fostered inequality (Solomon 1971). Confucianism was attacked for its emphasis on hierarchical relations between all people, dependence on authority figures, avoidance of conflict, and knowing one's proper place in the larger order of the world. Mao rejected these values and norms and vigorously advocated new modes of interaction and the creation of a new, egalitarian society (Hinton 1966, Whyte 1974). Contrary to these ideals, one of the major conclusions of our study is that hierarchical authority relations and paternalism continue to characterize almost every unit relationship (leader-staff, professional-auxiliary personnel, doctor-patient, and the consultations between leaders and professionals at different levels). Avoidance of conflict also persists. Although the nature of assignment to the unit forces people to deal with each other and to resolve rather than avoid problems, conflict seems to be handled indirectly.

Life in the units retains many similarities to descriptions of life in China before 1949, notably the importance of the family and of personal relations (*ganqing*) in interactions with nonkin (Fried 1953). Deference to authority, conflict avoidance, and the use of third-party intermediaries to resolve disputes are also traditional cultural behavioral patterns (Solomon 1971, Lubman 1967). Finally, although local-level leaders in prerevolutionary China operated with considerably more autonomy, the conception of their role and the source of their authority were similar to those of unit leaders today. Leaders, especially party leaders, are expected to set a good example for their constituencies. Like the Confucian scholar-official (*zhunzi*) ideal, their authority depends on their moral character and can be challenged should the masses judge it necessary.

Also striking are the similarities to behavior in Chinese organizations outside the People's Republic. For example, in a study of management practices in Taiwan, Silin (1976) observed the following characteristics: management is highly centralized; executives often hold multiple posts; there is a tendency to withhold information; there is little horizontal communication; and people believe that personal relationships are more effective than formal relationships. Meetings, too, serve much the same purpose that they do in a *danwei*.

> There are a variety of ways in which executives learn the line. Meetings are particularly important. In Taiwan meetings, especially when the boss is present, serve many purposes but they are too public to discuss and resolve serious issues or problems. Prohibitions against the expression of alternative views mean that even meetings held specifically to resolve problems are unlikely to do so. Meetings rather involve communication, particularly downward, and status definition. (Silin 1976, 75)

One of Silin's informants explained the difficulty of expressing views directly.

> "In the company, or maybe even in China in general, this [inability to express opposing views] is our biggest weakness . . . , for people will not speak out but will prefer to talk to the person who leads a meeting after it is over. This a question of face. They are afraid [*pa*] of the leader. They do not want to hurt the quality of their relationship [*ganqing*] with the other members of the group." (Ibid., 69–70)

There are, of course, considerable differences between organizational behavior in China and Taiwan, most of which can be linked to their different political and economic systems. Thus it is not suprising that the position of the boss in a Taiwan enterprise is far more autonomous than that of a work unit leader. On the other hand, assertive behavior by subordinates, though often indirect, seems to be more genuinely acceptable in work units.[2]

Overall, it appears that the structural characteristics of the unit system

2. Silin (1976) argues that in Taiwan enterprises, criticism from below is often viewed as negative or even devious. Our observations indicate an acceptance of criticism both in ritualized form and in the indirect mechanisms of feedback to higher levels.

reinforce traditional dependent modes of interaction. Units are part of an administrative system that takes most individual initiative away from job assignment, from moving once a job is obtained, and from many daily work and home decisions. Most of one's needs can be met, and often *must* be met, by the unit. The members' heightened dependence on the unit and isolation from other units reinforces their dependence on authority figures within the unit. Unit leaders themselves are part of authority hierarchies that tie all units to the central government.

These structural characteristics of the work unit system may have facilitated the occurrence and perpetuation of the Cultural Revolution, a social movement that made work units more controlling than before or since.[3] During the Cultural Revolution, "people-processing" (Goffman 1961) as an organizational goal became the highest priority. Although work goals necessarily continued to be met in the hospital, in the medical college they were abandoned for several years while staff and former leaders were reeducated. The replacement of *danwei* leaders by others who were politically acceptable (but often not as professionally competent) increased the distance between staff and leaders. In this setting, physicians avoided offering opinions, and in general, people were reluctant to rely on either indirect or group voice to express dissatisfaction, for fear of being criticized on political grounds. The tactics employed during the Cultural Revolution to reeducate (or "process") the unit staff were strikingly similar to those employed in total institutions such as asylums or prisons. People were removed from familiar ties, often even from their families. In countless compulsory meetings, they were subjected to the pressure of peers and those judged ideologically correct, and in some cases to physical humiliation.

This build-up of control was accomplished in part because it was directed by the party, or by factions in the party, which exercised authority over all unit affairs; in part because the staff population within units could not readily leave and find work elsewhere; in part because the passive system of control already in place in units provided entrée into both the work and the private life of staff members; and in part because channels of appeal are more easily frustrated when one is denied membership in overlapping institutions. The feedback mechanisms and delicate controls over unit lead-

3. The information we obtained about events during the Cultural Revolution is retrospective and limited by the biases inherent in the participant-observation methodology (see appendix 7). Nevertheless, because we were in China during a moderate phase and people were being encouraged to criticize the Cultural Revolution, the accounts given us are probably more reliable than those gathered before 1976.

ership that we observed were not sufficiently institutionalized to counter this encroachment. Even the position of unit leaders was too fragile to provide a basis for resistance.

Very recently, in an attempt to limit the extent of control by units over their members, the regime has instituted reforms to undercut the power of the party and to introduce more individual input into management and job assignment (Pepper 1981, Pepper 1982, Wei 1980, Hu 1981). These reforms may alter the combination of characteristics in the unit system, and the structural context that made it such a powerful instrument of control from 1966 to 1976.

Given the persistence of traditional cultural values and behavioral norms within Chinese organizations, is it legitimate to label the *danwei* a traditional institution? Western authors have tended to postulate convergence of modernizing nations along a model carved out by the West, with diverging characteristics labeled "traditional." For example, until recently the Japanese organizational traits of permanent employment and personal loyalty to the company have been defined as not modern or efficient (Cole 1979). The case of Japan demonstrates clearly that modernity and efficiency cannot be defined only in terms of a break with all traditional norms and values or an imitation of the Western model of development. Rather, one must begin with a definition of progress established by the nation itself. For China, two sometimes conflicting goals explain many of its struggles since 1949: economic development and socialist egalitarianism.

The Chinese revolution transformed the institutions of a preindustrial, agrarian economy through the implementation of land reform, gradual collectivization of agriculture, socialization of industry and commerce, and central direction of investment and planning. Although industry has developed and there has been overall economic growth, shifts in policies and major political turmoil have prevented steady development (Howe 1978). On the local level, the organization of workplaces into units and the control over distribution and assignment of workers have promoted stable development. Initially, this system helped integrate the population into a national economy by linking all workplaces with the national economic plan and establishing a system of communication among various levels of leadership.

On the other hand, several characteristics of the *danwei* system seem to obstruct efficient economic development. One of these is the position the unit occupies in the overall structure of society. Isolated from other, comparable units, the *danwei* is dependent on a vertical authority reminiscent of a feudal estate. Within the unit, and between the unit and higher levels, relationships are deferential. Dependency is heightened by the lack of alternatives for employment outside the unit—for staff *and* leaders—and by the extent of the organization's influence over both work and personal life. During the early years of the Communist revolution this form of economic self-reliance was functional and even essential for survival,[4] but today such isolation hinders coordination of activities among units engaged in similar enterprises. Because information and authority is vertical, communication between units may be delayed and a sense of competition rather than cooperation fostered. Although these characteristics may not be overwhelming disadvantages for some sectors of the economy, they may handicap efficient progress in planning and research and the development of large-scale industry. This problem may also impede progress in biomedical research or the transfer of information useful for patient care.

A second deterrent to economic development is the limited real authority of local-level unit leaders, who operate cautiously under the supervision of both higher levels and watchful staff members.[5] The unit system is not the sole cause of unit leaders' conservative behavior; the shifting political winds in China during the past three decades have produced a cautious attitude among all who must take responsibility for actions that might leave them vulnerable to future criticism. Risk taking under such circumstances is minimal. The unit system perpetuates passivity in leaders' responses to challenge and offers them few opportunities for individual initiative.

Finally, the Chinese themselves have acknowledged the negative effects of units' "ownership" of staff, particularly in the case of intellectuals (Hu 1981). State-controlled assignment to work units has had the positive results of restricting migration to urban areas and providing stability in labor-force allocation plans—feats rarely accomplished by other developing nations, even those with far fewer people in the labor force. Nevertheless, the system of permanent employment in units has not rewarded its members with predictable promotions or pay raises. On the contrary, the best-educated, most skilled, and senior staff have been the least mobile. People have not been rewarded in accordance with either "rational" criteria such as skills or education, as Western organizations profess to do, or the more "traditional" criteria of age, which has been applied in Japan (Clark 1979). The unpre-

---

4. The comparison with pre-1949 economic strategies was suggested by William A. Fischer (personal communication).

5. Bernstein (1982, 260) has suggested that the *danwei* leader is a modern version of the clan leader of traditional China. Although there are some similiarities, our data do not support the analogy.

dictability of the Chinese system has had a negative effect on unit members' motivation, satisfaction, and probably loyalty, and contrasts sharply with the socialist vision of workers "owning" their workplaces.

What of the second goal of the Chinese regime, that of socialist egalitarianism? Here again, the *danwei* system appears to offer both reinforcement and resistance.

The usual indicators of status differentials reveal continuing inequities, but also a general leveling process in comparison with pre-1949 China. Housing in our unit is limited, with most families receiving more or less equivalent facilities, and the size of housing does not seem closely related to occupational status. On the other hand, there is a sixfold difference in income between the lowest- and highest-paid staff members. These differences, however, are often offset by the effects of combined family income and by the provision of critical services for all unit members regardless of income: free medical coverage, retirement benefits, maternity benefits, inexpensive child care (which promotes female employment and thus increases family income levels), and some small redistribution of funds during holidays. Educational opportunities are available to all unit children through secondary school, with competitive examinations and continuing education classes established to rectify Cultural Revolution losses, although this competition may eventually increase status differences. Finally, private cars are forbidden, except for use by the medical college president. Travel and other entertainment opportunities are limited. Rationing of cloth, some food items, and many consumer goods keeps unit members dressing, eating, and buying similarly.

The unit is far from ultraegalitarian. Differences exist in occupation, income, education, and some benefits, especially between ordinary workers or lower-level personnel and administrators or professionals. Furthermore, between members of different work units and between urban and rural citizens, income differentials are substantial. In our unit, however, there is no visible accumulation of privilege, and we observed constraints on middle-level cadres as well as evidence of their power.[6] Overall, distribution of the basic necessities of life appears far more equitable in today's *danwei* than in pre-1949 China.

Yet if we enlarge the definition of socialist egalitarianism to include the tendency to perpetuate or erode traditional, nonegalitarian values and

6. Some of the perquisites of high-level cadres, however, are impressive. These include much higher incomes, access to privileges such as the special ward in our hospital, and private use of unit cars (Butterfield 1981a).

norms of behavior, then our observations suggest that units may be a conservative force. As discussed earlier in this section, the more traditional patterns of relationships seem to have persisted even during the Cultural Revolution. Within the hospital, the breakdown in supervision may be viewed as a trend away from traditional reliance on authority relations, but it does not appear to have increased the independence of unit members. Rather, it seems to have generated confusion, fear, and perhaps even greater dependency in uncertain times. In fact dependency on authority figures, avoidance of direct conflict, and the use of traditional devices by unit staff, leaders, and clients to make their ways in the unit world may even have been exaggerated by the Cultural Revolution experience.

Thus, in China, following a socialist revolution that redistributed ownership in agriculture and industry, a variety of new political, economic, and social institutions were created. In our work unit, however, we observed a microcosm of a society that is at once revolutionary and traditional. The persistence of these contradictions indicates the difficulty of transforming a society's values and institutions. China's establishment of a socialist economic base has not automatically dictated a new set of social relations.

DANWEI *AND THE MODERNIZATION OF MEDICINE*

Since the end of the Cultural Revolution, China has reordered priorities in health care, with emphasis on medical research, advanced technology, and development of urban medical centers (Lampton 1981). At the same time, health planners have become concerned about cost containment and improving the quality of primary care for the rural population, issues faced by most other developing nations (Wu 1981).

Recent policy decisions seem directed at achieving a balance between excellent medical education and tertiary care on the one hand and attention to rural needs on the other, and at deciding on the best mechanism for achieving modernization. Even though it is recognized that individual effort is responsible for many advances, Chinese authorities and researchers alike have been reluctant to promote individual attention. Instead, the emphasis has been on the importance of team effort, perhaps best exemplified in descriptions of the synthesis of insulin by Chinese scientists (Horn 1969). In our unit, many of our friends and colleagues avoided individual reward for special efforts, no matter how difficult or successful. Yet their frequent discussion of this issue indicates that individual recognition may in fact be quite important to them.

In the United States, medical institutions compete for talented professionals. "Soft" grant money awarded through national competition (such as National Institutes of Health awards) is movable and represents a concrete benefit (in terms of both prestige and financial gain) to any institution able to lure a successful physician or researcher from his home base. Therefore, if an institution sees a need for a special type of physician or a new skill, it initiates a vigorous attempt to recruit from outside. Disadvantages of this system include the professional and personal trauma associated with frequent relocation and the damage done to the institution that previously nurtured the professional. Furthermore, under this system institutions with the resources that support recruitment continue to improve at the expense of those that are less well-to-do.

In sharp contrast, Chinese medical units are remarkably stable. The professional staff are a resource not easily released. If demand arises for a new procedure, technology, or skill, the most typical organizational response is to train and promote an internal candidate. Thus, advancement within the system may depend on being chosen to learn a new skill and may lead to personal gain and increased professional autonomy. Although this system avoids the difficulties observed in the United States, it too has several disadvantages. The candidates selected may lack an appropriate or sufficient background, especially when political criteria play a prominent role in job selection, as they did during the Cultural Revolution. Professionals may also feel ambivalence about promotion, because the trauma of the Cultural Revolution was visited most severely on the more aggressive, well-educated professionals. It is clear that these events have not been forgotten.

Another disadvantage is the inability of the Chinese professional to use relocation as a bargaining chip. In the U.S. job market, the home institution may make a counteroffer to avoid losing its resource, and these counteroffers allow advancement or improvements in work conditions. Chinese units do not appear to be under similar pressures.

Finally, a perhaps predictable problem has arisen as more and more Chinese physicians seek training in Western countries. Physicians who have taken part in programs in the United States or Western Europe may return to their work units unable to utilize the skills or training they obtain. We met several physican-cum-scientists who had learned advanced research techniques or clinical skills but lacked the materials or equipment necessary to pursue their research. Perhaps increased flexibility for transfer will be allowed for those who acquire skills that can be utilized only in more sophisticated units, or a series of special units with increased lateral mobility for staff will be established. Such strategies, however, might reinforce a hierarchy of units contrary to the goal of socialist egalitarianism.

We have looked at China through the narrow window afforded by living for five months in a Chinese hospital *danwei*. Our observations suggest that the relationship between medical personnel and their work units will influence efficient incorporation of modern medical technologies and skills. The *danwei* system will play an important role as the regime faces the difficult tasks of modernizing medicine, distributing health care services, and containing costs.

Appendixes

The Nursing Shifts

Nine nurses and two head nurses are assigned to the infectious disease ward. The assignment of nurses to the various shifts is as follows.

Day Shift [Generally six nurses are on duty.]

Two or three nurses are assigned to the nursing shift each week—one or two to the early morning shift, 8:00 A.M.–4:00 P.M. and one to the 10:00 A.M.–6:00 P.M. shift.

Two nurses are assigned to the treatment shift each week—one to the early morning shift and one to the 10:00–6:00 shift.

One nurse is assigned to the chief shift (overseeing the treatment shift) each day.

The nurses rotate covering the period from noon to 2:00 P.M., when the other staff take naps or rest.

Night Shift [Generally two nurses are on duty sequentially.]

One nurse is assigned to the evening shift (5:30 P.M.–1:30 A.M.), a different nurse each evening.

One nurse is assigned to the night shift (1:30–8:30 A.M.), a different nurse each night.

The head nurses rotate their duties during the day (8:00–4:00 and 10:00–6:00), as well as taking turns with night duty.

RESPONSIBILITIES OF EACH NURSING SHIFT

Items listed on a chart in the nursing station of the infectious disease ward of the Second Attached Hospital of Hubei Provincial Medical College:

The 10:00–6:00 Shift

1. 10:00 A.M.: Come to work, check all equipment, etc. Learn condition of critical patients.
2. 11:00 A.M.: Eat lunch. 11:30: Return from lunch.
3. Make rounds. Ask patients to rest at noon hour. Make frequent rounds and watch all IV fluids. Lock all ward doors.
4. Wash hats and masks and medicine cups, and put all these items into sterilizer [the cabinet in the nursing station in which aerosolized formaldehyde is sprayed].
5. Prepare medicines for afternoon treatment.
6. Measure 2:00 P.M. temperatures of all patients.
7. 4:00 P.M.: Distribute all medicine by mouth.
8. Change bedding for patients who have been discharged and sterilize this and count it. Write on blackboard that patient has been discharged, that bedding was counted, etc.
9. Go to hospital pharmacy, take chart there to add up bill of patient to be discharged.
10. Change all injection instruments at supply department. Prepare all bottles, needles, dressings for evening shift.
11. Treat new patients and carry out physician orders regarding them.
12. Help pediatric patients who do not have relatives here to eat, wash feet, and take a bath. [This item does not usually apply to the ID ward, which generally does not admit children and where relatives of patients are rarely allowed.]
13. 3:00 P.M.: Open entrance door.
14. Write report and introduce conditions to evening shift nurses. Introduce critical patients' conditions at patients' bedside.

The Early Morning Shift [8:00 A.M.–4:00 P.M.]
[Note: Duties of the early morning and 10:00–6:00 shifts can be shared.]

1. In morning, do morning shift work [the nursing, treatment, or chief shift duties].
2. 11:00 A.M.: Go and eat. 11:30: Take up shift work. Receive new patients, critical patients, give transfusions.
3. Make rounds. Urge patients to have a rest. Lock doors.
4. Wash hats, masks, medicine cups, sterilize with steam.
5. Prepare medicines and instruments for afternoon treatment.
6. Measure temperatures at 2:00 P.M.
7. Clean steam sterilization cabinet.

8. Before leaving, introduce conditions to 10:00–6:00 shift, including treatment situations at all patients' beds, especially for critical patients.
9. 3:00 P.M.: Open entrance door.

Nursing Shift [General nursing duties are performed by nurses on all shifts.]

1. Count all equipment, bedding, clothing, thermometers, etc.
2. Ask the mildly ill patients to put bedding, cabinets, and mosquito net all in order, and to keep the ward clean. Collect all empty medicine bottles for sterilization.
3. Treat critical patients [help them eat, change soiled bedding].
4. Examine and record 10:00 A.M. temperature and pulse. Dysentery patients: also record twenty-four-hour stools.
5. Count all dirty bedding and clothes and get clean clothes from laundry.
6. Change sheets of patients who have been discharged and put cabinet [next to patient's bed] in order.
7. Help critical patients and children to eat meals, and wash bowls after meals.
8. Introduce critical patients' conditions to the early morning shift. Give them clean sheets.
9. Sterilize dirty bedding and clothes. Record number of sterilized bedding and clothes on blackboard.
10. Each day, send urine and stool samples twice: first before 10:30 A.M., second before 4:30 P.M.
11. Help critical patients and children to wash feet and bathe.
12. Sterilize masks and hats. Send out dirty ones to laundry and bring back clean ones.

Important Weekly Duties of Nursing Shift

1. Every fifteen days, change all bedding and clothes. Take them to the laundry.
2. Every Tuesday and Friday morning, clean steam sterilizer room.
3. Every Tuesday, Thursday, and Saturday, change the "contagion" white coats [used to see highly infectious patients].

Chief Shift

1. Hear about critically ill patients from night shift at morning report.
2. Call outpatient department and report number of empty beds.

3. Update patients' medicine cards [containing the physicians' medication orders]. Send the consult requests [*tongzhidan*] for all appropriate patients in infectious disease to be seen by specialists, get X rays, etc. Send orders for Chinese and Western medicine at the pharmacy.
4. Go and get medicine in medicine tray from the pharmacy. For those patients leaving the hospital, go get the medicine bill.
5. Give medicine to each patient. Make sure each really takes the medicine. Two nurses go to each patient and watch patient put it down.
6. Show new patients around the ward. Introduce the surroundings of the ward, the sterilization standards [where they can and cannot go, what the rules are, where to wash up, and so on].
7. Look around ward, understand conditions. Give report to next shift on each patient.

Important Weekly Duties of Chief Shift

1. Each Monday, Wednesday, and Saturday afternoon, check the patients' medicine cards to see if correct.
2. Once a week, check the emergency supply of medicines and make sure each patient gets what is ordered.
3. Each Wednesday and Saturday, check the fluid medicine by mouth that each patient takes. Make sure it is replenished every three days.

Treatment Shift

1. Count equipment [needles, IV tubes, and so on].
2. Carry out all treatment, including long term, short term, IVs, enemas, collect urine specimens—wash area, let urine come for a bit, collect some, let person finish urinating, all kinds of tests.
3. Prepare afternoon and next morning treatment equipment.
4. Sterilization room: Exchange used syringes for freshly sterilized ones. For night shift, prepare the IV bottles, syringes, needle tips, tubing for enemas, nose-stomach tubes, cotton swabs.
5. Clean treatment room.
6. Tell next shift what medicines the patients still need.

Important Weekly Duties of Treatment Shift

1. Each Monday, sterilize all the cotton swabs and dressings, tongue depressors, scissors, and replace sterilization fluid.
2. Empty wastebaskets twice a week.

Evening Shift [5:30 P.M.–1:30 A.M.]

1. Check equipment from previous shift. Write colored temperature chart. Check injection tubes, clothing, bedding, patients. For critical patients, the information should be exchanged at bedside.
2. Do all treatment and nursing duties of this shift.
3. At 7:00 P.M., summarize total fluid intake and output of patients.
4. At 8:00 P.M., prepare bed pans for critical patients. Put down mosquito net.
5. Prepare bottles, injection tubes, and needles for night shift.
6. Clean nursing station, treatment office, and staff washroom. Use ultraviolet rays to sterilize rooms. Wash towels, clean sink, add sterilization fluid in pans [used for hand sterilization].
7. Make rounds frequently to all wards in order to understand patient conditions.
8. Write in patient duty book ["ward diary"]. Clean up nursing station and desk drawers.
9. Check all transfusion medicine that day shift left.
10. Write evening shift report. Introduce conditions to night shift. Introduce critical patients at bedside.
11. 7:00 P.M.: Fetch milk. 8:00 P.M.: Ask visitors to leave. 9:30: Turn off lights and urge patients to sleep.

Important Weekly Duties of Evening Shift

1. On Wednesdays, check all medicines prepared for use, including injections and pills.
2. Change alcohol and other disinfectant that has been used to sterilize plastic needles.

Night Shift [1:30 A.M.–8:00 A.M.]

1. Come at 1:30 A.M.
2. Check all equipment—injections tubes, thermometers, etc.
3. Make rounds with the evening shift. Introduce each patient's condition at bedside.
4. Carry out all treatment and nursing duties of night shift.
5. Frequently make rounds and observe critical patients' conditions.
6. Receive new patients and do all for new patients that should be done.
7. 4:00 A.M.: Begin preparing IV solution and intramuscular injection. If there is a critical patient, schedule can be altered.

8. 6:00 A.M.: Take blood for lab tests before patient has breakfast.
9. Do the "Three Checks and the Three Corrects."
10. 8:00 A.M.: Give intramuscular injection and distribute medicines by mouth.
11. Count fluid intake and output for previous twenty-four hours.
12. Open entrance door.
13. Write night shift report and introduce conditions to next shift.

Schedule of Important Weekly Ward Nursing Duties

A chart appearing in the nursing station of the infectious disease ward of the Second Attached Hospital of Hubei Provincial Medical College:

Monday: Morning Report. Announce the week's work. Sterilize the pans used to treat patients. Change sterile fluids. Replace chart holders (if necessary), pails, thermometers, and any containers that receive tubes. Director of ward and head nurse will decide if relatives can see patients.

Tuesday: Change bedding (every two weeks). Afternoon: Political study meeting [*zhengzhi xuexi*] (half the nurses go each week).

Wednesday: Count the drugs in the drug table. Count the emergency medicine in storage. Organize and carry out the nursing rounds [*hushi chafang*]. Health aides sterilize bedpans, change sterile fluids used by health aides.

Thursday: Order ward properties, medicines. Sharpen needle tips.

Friday: Count properties. Be aware of relatives on ward. Cut fingernails of critically ill patients, wash their hair, change their clothes (in addition to changing whenever else it is needed), and other basic nursing tasks. Afternoon: Study sessions [*zhiwu xuexi*].

Saturday: Sum up week's work, whether it has been done well or not. Afternoon: Clean up, inside and outside.

OTHER PERIODIC EVENTS

1. Once a month: Patients, nurses, and physicians have meeting to exchange opinions, one to two hours.
2. Twice a month: Head nurse and director of ward have meeting to arrange work of ward.

3. Once a month: Storage of deliveries of supplies [soap, towels, mops, and so on].
4. Once a month: All physicians and nurses in internal medicine and infectious disease have meeting, discuss work, praise good workers.
5. Once a month: Count all properties of ward, done by one nurse and head nurse.
6. Each day: Change isolation clothing [sterile gowns].
7. Every Monday, Wednesday, and Friday: Help patients to buy things [snacks, toilet articles, and so on].

Weekly Schedule of the Infectious Disease Ward Head Nurse

A chart appearing in the nursing station of the infectious disease ward of the Second Attached Hospital of Hubei Provincial Medical College:

Monday: Morning Report 8:00. Arrange week's special work, including anything specially ordered from the administration [which the head nurse has learned about at hospital meetings]. Inspect work of nurses, whether done well or poorly. Inspect the three levels of patients [that is, enforce the care required of these levels. The physicians assign patients to the three levels: critical patients (nurses do everything, patients do not move), medium (nurses help, do not do all), light (patient does everything for himself, is just there to rest)]. Inspect who goes in to see "critical" patients. Make sure wards are clean and relatives kept out.

Afternoon: If there is no need to contact people outside the infectious disease ward, then go to meetings.

Tuesday: Accompany head of infectious disease ward on morning rounds. Inspect medical treatment responsibilities. Inspect charts to see they are up-to-date, tests done well and recorded. Inspect patients' conditions. Prepare to give own rounds for the nurses on patient care.

Afternoon: Political study meetings.

Wednesday: Organize nurses' rounds. Inspect nurses' sterile and sanitary conditions. Inspect how the health aides carry out their work.

Afternoon: Inspect and correct the parts of charts for which nurses are responsible. Inspect the distribution of medicine (head nurse responsible for correct amount). Inspect quality of chart work [graphs, arranging tests, and so on].

Thursday: Inspect emergency medicines, materials, and equipment. Inspect the "Five Rules of Medicine": (1) location, (2) quantity, (3) quality, (4) use, (5) who is in charge of the medicine. Inspect the property of the ward [for repairs, theft, and so on].
Afternoon: Submit list of ward's needs to maintenance and supplies department.

Friday: Accompany head of ward on rounds. Inspect important shift duties. Inspect patient conditions.
Afternoon: Study period.

Saturday: Morning Report: Sum up week's work. Check to see if system has been carried out. Make example of good people, good work. Point out still existing problems. Inspect student nurses' education.
Afternoon: Clean up [physicians, nurses, health aides all together].

Service Slogans for Medical Personnel

A chart appearing in the nursing station of the infectious disease ward of the Second Attached Hospital of Hubei Provincial Medical College:

ESTABLISH THE FOUR ATTITUDES AND THE FOUR STRICTNESSES OF MEDICAL WORK STYLE

Four Attitudes [Sixin]

Warmly receive the patient.
Examine the patient carefully.
Treat the patient seriously.
Explain things patiently.

Four Strictnesses [Siyen]

Strictly carry out your duties.
Do all tasks seriously.
Strictly check up on all things.
Carry out rules strictly.

IN THE PATIENT AREAS, REQUIRE THE THREE SOFTS AND THE SIX DON'TS

Three Softs [Sanching]

Speak softly.
Walk gently.
Treat the patient gently.

Six Don'ts [Liubu]

No stoves or raw vegetables can be brought into ward.
Patients and visitors cannot read charts without permission.
Don't make large noises in the ward.
Visitors and relatives of patients should not lie down or sleep in patients' beds.
No smoking, no spitting.
No littering, either out of window or on the ground.

FOR MEDICAL PERSONNEL ON DUTY: "THE FIVE NOT ALLOWED"

Five Not Allowed [Wubuzhun]

Not allowed to come late or leave early.
No absences without permission.
Not allowed to leave while on duty.
Not allowed to conduct private affairs while on duty.
Don't put off today's work until tommorow.

Continuing Education for Nurses

In addition to lectures for nurses given in the hospital and classes held for nurses preparing for the examination for promotion, lectures for nurses were held around the city on Fridays. The following is a typical notice for a Friday afternoon lecture.

THE CHINESE ACADEMY OF NURSING, WUHAN BRANCH:
SCHEDULE OF SPECIAL MEETINGS

November 1979 Topics

1. "Common Causes of Coma, Differentiating Degrees and Appropriate Nursing Care"
2. "Definitions and Physiology of Premature Births and Treatment of Common, Serious Complications"
   "Clinical Manifestations of Intracranial Hemorrhage, Principles of Treatment, Differential Diagnosis and Nursing Care"
3. "Manifestations of Hepatic Cirrhosis and Common Complications, and Correct Nursing Care for Patients with Ascites"
   "Predisposing Factors of Liver Coma: Early Stage Diagnosis and Nursing Care"
4. "Newborn Bilirubin Metabolism Characteristics, Common Manifestations of Jaundice and Other Common Diseases during the Newborn Period, Uniting Several Different Treatments and Nursing Care"
5. "What Is Acute Pulmonary Edema? Principles to Understand: The Causal Mechanisms, Clinical Manifestations, Emergency Principles, Giving Oxygen to Edema Patients Who Develop Emphysema"

Duties of the Health Aides

DAILY ROUTINE OF HEALTH AIDES

6:30 A.M.   Pour water for patients (get boiled water for patients' thermoses), help patients get meals, then go home for breakfast at 8:00. [Getting the patients' food involves going to the patients' kitchen behind the hospital and pulling the metal cart with the food inside from the kitchen to the ward, then dishing out the food to the patients.]

8:30 A.M.   Mop ward floors, order daily food for patients, clean bathrooms; in spare time, help nurses make cotton swabs, record temperature charts, in patients' charts, etc.

11:00 A.M. Go and get food for patients.

11:30 A.M. Go home for lunch and rest (noon–3:00).

3:00 P.M.   Come back, pour water, clean, dust, help nurses.

4:30 P.M.   Go and get food for patients, help patients with food.

5:30 P.M.   Go home.

WEEKLY SCHEDULE OF HEALTH AIDES

A chart appearing in the nursing station of the infectious disease ward of the Second Attached Hospital of Hubei Provincial Medical College:

Monday   Clean the ward and the mosquito nets. Sweep the grounds. Sweep under bedside tables and dust the radiators.

Tuesday   Mop the corridor, floors, walls, and corners. [Political study is not required for workers. These workers rotate attendance.]

Wednesday   Sterilize bedpans. Change sterilization fluid.

164

Thursday	Take day off in turn. [The three health aides rotate three rest days: Thursday, Saturday, and Sunday.]
Friday	Mop the food dropoff room, the bedpan room, the bathroom, and the bathtub. Dust the windows.
Saturday	Take day off in turn. Count basins [for face washing], bedpans, spitoons, and other ward properties.
Sunday	Take day off in turn.
Daily Work	Sweep floor, bring food to patients, mop floor on days besides Tuesdays, help patients to buy small toilet articles, do things for patients, help nurses.

Methodology

This study is based on a five-month period of participant-observation and informant interviewing. Within this period we also conducted a three-month study of patients on the infectious disease ward, which involved simple enumeration and sampling techniques as well as interviewing. Our initial role within the hospital *danwei* was as representatives of Yale University School of Medicine. One of us, as the physician, was viewed as the major figure involved in planning the medical exchange program. However, as the other took on a full-time English teaching position, her status within the hospital and medical college rose dramatically because of the pressing need for English-language speakers in China today. Other important roles included being residents of the unit and parents of an infant who occasionally attended the unit day-care center but was from the outset known to all unit members.

In each of these roles, we were "participants as observers" (McCall and Simmons 1969, 35); that is, we participated fully in the life of the unit as acknowledged observers, although the objectives of our observation were not always explicitly defined. Each role gave us access to different experiences, information, and perspectives. We conducted informant interviewing both together and separately. Interviews ranged from formal meetings with medical college and hospital officials to informal conversations with friends, staff, and patients. The data used consisted of daily logs of events, impressions, conversations, and interviews, as well as systematic records kept on patients in the infectious disease ward.

The problems encountered in an ethnographic study such as this are difficult to avoid. First, in addition to the normal reactive effects of an observer's presence on the phenomena being observed, we were foreign observers. Foreign access to information about life in China is a highly sensitive issue for all Chinese citizens. (Even among the Chinese themselves, access to information defines one's status in society.) We attempted to check on informant credibility by asking the same questions of several people. The longer we lived in China, the more sure we became of the reliability, or lack of reliability, of our observations. Yet the problem will never be eliminated.

We learned about the history of relationships among *danwei* staff during the past three decades only gradually, and our information was at best incomplete. Among the actors were old enemies and old friends, complex networks including a multiplicity of statuses and roles, and formal and informal relationships. In a setting such as this, staging and choreographed devices effectively mask interpersonal relations; and the ritual and ceremony that clearly persist in China today make it even harder to identify "who" people are (Renée C. Fox, personal communication).

A second difficulty typical of our methodology was exaggerated by the location of this study. Life in a work unit is intense. Socialization forces operate upon all who participate, including foreign participant-observers. The potential for getting too involved with the people, called over-rapport, was ever present, and was intensified by our multiple entry into unit life. Of course, our involvement in the unit was also the very substance of the study itself, providing the detail and the flavor needed to convey what it is like to live there.

Complicating the difficulties that characterize field research is our concern for protecting our friends and colleagues in this *danwei* from negative repercussions that might result from our published observations. We were in China during a period of political relaxation; yet since we returned to the United States, contacts between Chinese and foreigners living in China have once again fallen under suspicion by Chinese authorities. We do not believe our depiction of the hospital as an example of the *danwei* is inflammatory or in any sense an exposé. Nevertheless, to protect the identities of our informants, we have not supplied detailed personal histories or detailed accounts of their experiences during the Cultural Revolution except when those details are crucial to an understanding of the dynamics of the unit.

Finally, any participant-observation study is inherently limited to being a *case study*: it is not representative. We do not know how typical our unit is of all hospitals or units in China. On the basis of information from Whyte and Parish (1983), we suspect that our unit resembles an "urban village" environment more than some, mainly because it is fairly large and the majority of staff live there and take advantage of the many services offered. This study, however, can report with confidence only on the social processes occurring within one *danwei* in China. Conclusions about the frequency of events in units, characteristics, behaviors, or attitudes must await the application of more systematic research methods.

Despite its drawbacks, the methodology of qualitative research was by far the best suited to our situation. It was not possible to go to China armed with a defined topic and all contingencies calculated in advance. The final thesis is a result of our immersion in the setting and our impressions of its most salient characteristics. We went through several stages of research. First we tried to learn as much as possible about our environment. We were introduced to the unit by the sponsorship of middle-level leaders, and we were accepted gradually by the people with whom we lived and worked, as well as by higher-level authorities. The quality of our data changed as we became more comfortable asking different questions. Several times, we reviewed and discussed all the material to reorient ourselves to theoretical issues and to generate new questions to ask. Most important, the analysis remained fluid. This freedom is the essence of the participant-observation method.

Bibliography

Abel-Smith, Brian. "Major Patterns of Financing and Organization of Medical Care in Countries Other Than the United States." In *Social Policy for Health Care*. New York: New York Academy of Medicine, 1969.

Aday, L. A., and Anderson, Robert. "Insurance Coverage and Access: Implications for Health Policy." *Health Services Research* 13 (1978): 369–77.

Allen, James B. *The Company Town in the American West*. Norman: University of Oklahoma Press, 1966.

Anderson, E. N. "Chinese Methods of Dealing with Crowding." *Urban Anthropology* 1 (1972): 141–50.

Anderson, Odin W. *Health Care: Can There Be Equity? The United States, Canada, and England*. New York: John Wiley and Sons, 1972.

Anderson, R., and Newman, J. F. "Societal and Individual Determinants of Medical Care in the United States." *Milbank Memorial Fund Quarterly* 51 (1973):95.

A Barefoot Doctor's Manual: The American Translation of the Official Chinese Paramedical Manual. Philadelphia: Running Press, 1977.

Barnett, A. Doak. *Cadres, Bureaucracy, and Political Power in Communist China*. New York: Columbia University Press, 1967.

———, ed. *Chinese Communist Politics in Action*. Seattle: University of Washington Press, 1969.

Barry, Brian. Review of *Exit, Voice, and Loyalty*, by Albert O. Hirschman. *British Journal of Political Science* 4 (January 1974):79–107.

Bates, Barbara. "Doctors and Nurses: Changing Roles and Relations." In *Dominant Issues in Medical Sociology*, edited by Howard D. Schwartz and Cary S. Kart. Reading, Mass.: Addison-Wesley, 1978.

Beijing Review 22, no. 41 (12 October 1979):6; 22, no. 47 (23 November 1979): 6–7; 23, no. 6 (11 February 1980):7; 24, no. 37 (14 September 1981):3; 24, no. 39 (28 September 1981):3; 25, no. 25 (28 July 1982):3.

Berg, Robert L.; Brooks, M. R., Jr.; and Savičevič, Miomir. *Health Care in Yugoslavia and the United States*. U.S. Department of Health, Education and Welfare Publication No. (NIH) 75-911. Bethesda, Md.: Fogarty International Center, National Institutes of Health, 1976.

Bernstein, Richard. *From the Center of the Earth: The Search for the Truth about China*. Boston: Little, Brown, 1982.

Bernstein, Thomas P. *Up to the Mountains and Down to the Villages*. New Haven: Yale University Press, 1977.

Birch, A. H. "Economic Models in Political Science: The Case of 'Exit, Voice, and Loyalty.'" *British Journal of Political Science* 5 (January 1975): 65–82.

Blecher, Marc, and White, Gordon. *Basic Level Politics in Contemporary China: A Technical Unit during and after the Cultural Revolution*. White Plains, N.Y.: M. E. Sharpe, 1980.

Blendon, Robert J. "Can China's Health Care Be Transplanted without Chinese Economic Policies?" *New England Journal of Medicine* 300 (1979): 1453–58.

———. "Public Health versus Personal Medical Care: The Dilemma of Post-Mao China." *New England Journal of Medicine* 304 (1981):981–82.

Bowers, John Z. *Western Medicine in a Chinese Palace: Peking Union College, 1917–1951*. New York: Josiah Macy, Jr., Foundation, 1974.

Bowers, John Z., and Purcell, Elizabeth, eds. *Medicine and Society in China*. New York: Josiah Macy, Jr., Foundation, 1974.

Broyelle, Claudio; Broyelle, Jacques; and Tschirhart, Evelyne. *China: A Second Look*. Atlantic Highlands, N.J.: Humanities Press, 1980.

Butterfield, Fox. *China: Alive in a Bitter Sea*. New York: Times Books, 1982.

———. "China, for a Fortunate Few at the Top, Is Paradise of Privilege and Perquisites." *New York Times*, 2 January 1981a, A6.

———. "China Ginerly Gives Private Business a Try." *New York Times*, 8 March 1981b, E3.

———. "Getting a Hotel Room in China: You're Nothing without a Unit." *New York Times*, 31 October 1979, C17.

Carleton, Wendy. *In Our Professional Opinion*. Notre Dame, Ind.: University of Notre Dame Press, 1978.

Cheng, T. O. "A View of Modern Chinese Medicine." *Annals of Internal Medicine* 78 (1973):285–90.

Cheng, T. O.; Axelrod, L.; and Leaf, A. "Medical Education and Practice in the People's Republic of China." *Annals of Internal Medicine* 83 (1975): 716–24.

"China and the United States Conclude Science and Technology, Cultural Accords." *China Exchange Newsletter* 7 (January 1979):3.

Clark, Rodney. *The Japanese Company*. New Haven: Yale University Press, 1979.

Cohen, M. S. "Epidemic Hemorrhagic Fever Revisited." *Reviews in Infectious Diseases* 4, no. 5 (September–October 1982):992–97.

Cohen, M. S.; Casals, J.; Hsiung, G.-D.; Kwei, H.-E.; Chin, C.-C.; Ge, H.-C.; Hsiang, C.-M.; Lee, P.-W.; Gibbs, C. J., Jr.; Gajdusek, D. C. "Epidemic Hemorrhagic Fever in Hubei Province, the People's Republic of China: A Clinical and Seriological Study." *Yale Journal of Biology and Medicine* 54 (1981):41–55.

Cole, Robert E. *Work, Mobility, and Participation: A Comparative Study of American and Japanese Industry*. Berkeley: University of California Press, 1979.

Committee on Scholarly Communication with the People's Republic of China. *Report of the Medical Delegation to the People's Republic of China*. Washington, D.C.: National Academy of Sciences, 1973.

Coser, Ruth L. "Authority and Decision-making in a Hospital: A Comparative Analysis." *American Sociological Review* 23 (1958):36–63.

Croizier, Ralph. *Traditional Medicine and Modern China: Science, Nationalism, and the Tensions of Cultural Change*. Cambridg , Mass.: Harvard University Press, 1968.

Davis-Friedmann, Deborah. "Retirement Practices in China: Recent Developments." Paper presented at the conference Aging and Retirement in Cross-Cultural Perspectives, Rockefeller Study and Conference Center, Bellagio, Italy, 22–26 June 1981.

Dimond, E. Grey. "Medical Education and Care in the People's Republic of China." *Journal of the American Medical Association*, no. 28 (6 December 1971):1552–57.

Dirschel, Kathleen M. "Teaching Nursing in China—An Exchange Program." *Nursing Outlook* 29, no. 12 (December 1981):722–26.

Eisenberg, J. M., and Williams, S. V. "Cost Containment and Changing Physicians' Practice Behavior." *Journal of the American Medical Association* 246 (13 November 1981):2195–2201.

Etzioni, Amitai. *A Comparative Analysis of Complex Organizations*. New York: Free Press, 1975.

Evans, J. R.; Hall, K. L.; and Warford, J. "Health Care in the Developing World: Problems of Scarcity and Choice." *New England Journal of Medicine* 305 (1981):1117–27.

Field, Mark G. *The Doctor and Patient in Soviet Russia*. Cambridge, Mass.: Harvard University Press, 1957.

Fischer, William A. "The Management of Industrial Science and Technology in the People's Republic of China: Opportunities and Problems." Paper presented at the Conference on Industrial Development in China, U.S. Department of Commerce, Washington, D.C., 24 February 1981.

Foreign Broadcast Information Service. *Daily Report of the People's Republic of China,* 9 September 1980, 3 November 1980, and 1 October 1981.

Fox, Renée C., and Swazey, Judith P. "Grandmother-Nurse and Nurse-Doctor: Portraits of Nursing in the People's Republic of China." Forthcoming.

Fraser, John. *The Chinese: Portrait of a People.* New York: Summit Books, 1980.

Freidson, Eliot. *Doctoring Together: A Study of Professional Control.* New York: Elsevier, 1975.

———. *Professional Dominance.* New York: Atherton Press, 1970a.

———. *The Profession of Medicine.* New York: Harper & Row, 1970b.

———, ed. *The Hospital in Modern Society.* New York: Free Press of Glencoe, 1963.

Freidson, Eliot, and Burford, Rhea. "Processes of Control in a Company of Equals." *Social Problems* 11 (Fall 1963):119–31.

Fried, Morton. *The Fabric of Chinese Society: A Study of the Social Life of a Chinese County Seat.* New York: Praeger, 1953.

Frolic, B. Michael. *Mao's People.* Cambridge, Mass.: Harvard University Press, 1980.

Garfield, Richard. "China's Nurses: Redefining Roles to Improve Health." *International Journal of Nursing Studies* 15, no. 3 (1978):129–34.

———. "Nursing Education in China." *Nursing Outlook* 26, no. 5 (May 1978):312–15.

Gish, Oscar. *Planning the Health Sector: The Tanzanian Experience.* New York: Holmes and Meier, 1975.

———. "Resource Allocation, Equality of Access, and Health." *International Journal of Health Services* 3 (1973):399–412.

Goffman, Erving. *Asylums: Essays on the Social Situation of Mental Patients and Other Inmates.* Garden City, N.Y.: Doubleday, Anchor Books, 1961.

Gold, Thomas B. "Back to the City: The Return of Shanghai's Educated Youth." *China Quarterly,* no. 84 (December 1980):55–70.

Goss, Mary E. W. "Influence and Authority among Physicians in an Outpatient Clinic." *American Sociological Review* 26 (February 1961):44.

———. "Patterns of Bureaucracy among Hospital Staff Physicians." In *The Hospital in Modern Society,* edited by Eliot Freidson. New York: Free Press of Glencoe, 1963.

Greene, Ruth A. *Hsiang-Ya Journal.* Hamden, Conn.: Shoe String Press, 1977.

Greenfield, Harry. *Allied Health Manpower: Trends and Prospects.* New York: Columbia University Press, 1969.

Gross, Glenn. "Professions, Markets, and Organizations." Manuscript.

Haug, Marie, and Lavin, Bebe. "Practitioner or Patient—Who's in Charge?" *Journal of Health and Social Behavior* 22 (September 1981): 212–28.

Haug, Marie, and Sussman, M. B. "Professional Autonomy and the Revolt of the Client." *Social Problems* 17 (Fall 1969):153–61.

"Health Care and the People's Republic of China." Report of a study tour co-sponsored by the University of Michigan–Dearborn and Michigan State University, 2–19 August 1979.

Henderson, G. E., and Cohen, M. S. "Are Biomedical Exchange Programs inside the People's Republic of China Feasible? Report of a Six-Month Study at Hubei Provincial Medical College." *Yale Journal of Biology and Medicine* 54 (1981):11–20.

———. "Health Care in the People's Republic of China: A View from Inside the System." *American Journal of Public Health* 72 (November 1982): 1238–45.

Hinman, A. R., and Parker, R., eds. "Health Services in Shanghai County." Supplement to *American Journal of Public Health* 72 (1982).

Hinton, William. *Fanshen: A Documentary of Revolution in a Chinese Village.* New York: Monthly Review Press, 1966.

Hirschman, Albert O. *Exit, Voice, and Loyalty.* Cambridge, Mass.: Harvard University Press, 1970.

Horn, Joshua. *Away with All Pests.* New York: Monthly Review Press, 1969.

Howe, Christopher. *China's Economy.* New York: Basic Books, 1978.

Hsu, Robert C. "The Barefoot Doctors of the People's Republic of China—Some Problems." *Journal of the American Medical Association* 218 (6 December 1971):124–27.

Hu, Ping. "On the Question of Intellectuals." *Beijing Review* 24, no. 7 (16 February 1981): 13–16.

Hu, T. W. "An Economic Analysis of the Cooperative Medical Services in the PRC." Washington, D.C.: Fogarty International Center, 1975.

Huang, C. S. "Medical Education in China." In *Medical Education in Asia: A Symposium.* New York: China Medical Board of New York, 1981.

Johnson, Terence J. *Professions and Power.* London: Macmillan, 1972.

Kleinman, Arthur, ed. *Medicine in Chinese Cultures.* U.S. Department of Health, Education and Welfare Publication No. (NIH) 75-653. Washington, D.C.: Geographic Health Studies, Fogarty International Center, 1975.

Kohn, Robert, and White, Kerr L. *Health Care, An International Study: Report of the World Health Organization Collaborative Study of Medical Care Utilization.* London: Oxford University Press, 1976.

Kolarska, Lena, and Aldrich, Howard. "Exit, Voice, and Silence: Consumers' and Managers' Responses to Organizational Decline." *Organizational Studies* 1 (1980):41–58.

Korzec, Michel, and Whyte, Martin K. "The Chinese Wage System." *China Quarterly*, no. 86 (June 1981): 248–73.

Knaus, William A. *Inside Russian Medicine: An American Doctor's First-Hand Report*. New York: Everest House, 1981.

Lampton, David M. "Changing Health Policy in the Post-Mao Era." *Yale Journal of Biology and Medicine* 54 (1981):21–26.

———. *Health, Conflict, and the Chinese Political System*. Ann Arbor: University of Michigan Center for Chinese Studies, 1974.

———. *The Politics of Medicine in China*. Boulder, Colo.: Westview Press, 1977.

Lasagna, Louis. "Herbal Pharmacology and Medical Therapy in the People's Republic of China." *Annals of Internal Medicine* 83, no. 6 (December 1975): 887–93.

Laver, Michael. "'Exit, Voice, and Loyalty' Revisited." *British Journal of Political Science* 6 (October 1976):463–82.

Lee, Rance P. "Chinese and Western Medical Care in China's Rural Communes: A Case Study." *Social Science and Medicine* 15A (March 1981):137–48.

Leys, Simon. *Chinese Shadows*. New York: Viking Press, 1977.

Lubman, Stanley. "Mao and Mediation: Politics and Dispute Resolution in Communist China." *California Law Review* 55 (November 1967):1284–1359.

Lyle, C. B. "Economic Irony and Cost Containment." *Annals of Internal Medicine* 90 (1979): 267–68.

"A Matchmaking Service." *Women of China*, April 1981, 39–40.

McCall, George J., and Simmons, J. L. *Issues in Participant Observation*. Reading, Mass.: Addison-Wesley, 1969.

McEwen, C. A. "Continuities in the Study of Total and Nontotal Institutions." *Annual Reviews in Sociology* 6 (1980):143–85.

Mechanic, David. *Politics, Medicine, and Social Science*. New York: John Wiley and Sons, 1974.

Mechanic, David, and Kleinman, Arthur. "Ambulatory Medical Care in the People's Republic of China: An Exploratory Study." *American Journal of Public Health* 70 (January 1980): 62–66.

Montagna, Paul D. *Occupations and Society*. New York: John Wiley and Sons, 1977.

Moore, M. E., and Berk, S. N. "Acupuncture for Chronic Shoulder Pain: An Experimental Study with Attention to the Role of Placebo and Hypnotic Susceptibility." *Annals of Internal Medicine* 84 (1976):381–84.

Munro, Donald J. *The Concept of Man in Contemporary China*. Ann Arbor: University of Michigan Press, 1979.

New, P. K., and New, M. L. "Reflections on Health Care in China: Lessons for the West." Paper presented at the conference Critical Issues in Health Care Delivery, University of Illinois, Chicago Circle, 10 June 1977.

Oi, Jean C. "State and Peasant in Contemporary China: The Politics of Grain Procurement." Ph.D. dissertation, University of Michigan, 1983.

Oksenberg, Michel. "Chinese Politics and the Public Health Issue." In *Medicine and Society in China*, edited by John Z. Bowers and Elizabeth Purcell. New York: Josiah Macy, Jr., Foundation, 1974.

———. "The Exit Pattern from Chinese Politics and Its Implications." *China Quarterly*, no. 67 (September 1976): 501.

Orleans, Leo. *Professional Manpower and Education in Communist China*. Washington, D.C.: National Science Foundation, 1961.

Parish, William L. "Egalitarianism in Chinese Society." *Problems of Communism* 30 (January–February 1981):37–53.

Parish, William L., and Whyte, Martin K. *Village and Family in Contemporary China*. Chicago: University of Chicago Press, 1978.

Parsons, Talcott. "The Sick Role and the Role of the Physician Reconsidered." *Milbank Memorial Fund Quarterly* 53 (1975):257–78.

———. *The Social System*. Glencoe, Ill.: The Free Press, 1951.

Pepper, Suzanne. "China's Universities: New Experiments in Socialist Democracy and Administrative Reform—A Research Report." *Modern China* 8 (April 1982):147–204.

———. "Chinese Universities: Experiments in Democracy." *Asian Wall Street Journal*, 2 September 1981, 8.

Quinn, Joseph R. *Medicine and Public Health in the People's Republic of China*. Washington, D.C.: U.S. Department of Health, Education and Welfare, Geographic Health Studies, Fogarty International Center, National Institutes of Health, 1972.

Reynolds, R. E. "Hospital Care." In U.S. Department of Health and Human Services, *Rural Health in the People's Republic of China*. National Institutes of Health Publication No. 812124. Washington, D.C., 1980.

Rosenthal, A. M. "Memories of a New China Hand." *New York Times Sunday Magazine*, 19 July 1981.

Rosenthal, Marilynn M. "Political Process and the Integration of Traditional and Western Medicine in the People's Republic of China." *Social Science and Medicine* 15A (September 1981):599–613.

Schurmann, Franz. *Ideology and Organization in Communist China*. Berkeley: University of California Press, 1966.

Schwartz, Howard D., and Kart, Cary S., eds. *Dominant Issues in Medical Sociology*. Reading, Mass.: Addison-Wesley, 1978.

Shehui Wenjiao Xingzheng Caiwu Zhidu Zhaibian [Excerpts on the system of social, cultural, and educational administration and finance]. Beijing: Chinese Finance and Economics Publishing House, 1979.

Shipp, Joseph C. "To Serve the People: Medical Education and Care in the People's Republic of China." *Annals of Internal Medicine* 97 (19 August 1982):277–79.

Shirk, Susan. "Recent Chinese Labor Policies and the Transformation of Industrial Organization in China." *China Quarterly* 88 (December 1981): 575.

Sidel, Ruth, and Sidel, Victor. *The Health of China*. Boston: Beacon Press, 1982.

Sidel, Victor W. "The Barefoot Doctors of the People's Republic of China." *New England Journal of Medicine* 286 (1972):1291–1300.

Sidel, Victor W., and Sidel, Ruth. *Serve the People: Observations on Medicine in the People's Republic of China*. New York: Josiah Macy, Jr., Foundation, 1973.

Silin, Robert H. *Leadership and Values: The Organization of Large-Scale Taiwanese Enterprises*. Cambridge, Mass.: Harvard University Press, 1976.

Skinner, William. "Marketing and Social Structure in Rural China." *Journal of Asian Studies* 24 (November 1964): 32–43.

Smith, Harvey L. "Two Lines of Authority Are One Too Many." *Modern Hospital* 84 (March 1955): 59–64.

Solomon, Richard H. *Mao's Revolution and the Chinese Political Culture*. Berkeley: University of California Press, 1971.

Stevens, Carl M. "Voice in Medical Markets: Consumer Participation." *Social Science Information* 13, no. 3 (1974): 33–48.

Stimson, Gary, and Webb, Barbara. *Going to See the Doctor*. London and Boston: Routledge and Kegan Paul, 1975.

Stinchcombe, Arthur L. "Organized Dependency Relations and Social Stratification." In *The Logic of Social Hierarchies*, edited by Edward O. Laumann, Paul M. Siegel, and Robert W. Hodge. Chicago: Markham, 1970.

Tien, H. Yuan. *China's Population Struggle*. Columbus: Ohio State University Press, 1973.

Twaddle, Andrew C. "Health Decisions and Sick Role Variations: An Exploration." *Journal of Health and Social Behavior* 10 (June 1969):105–15.

U.S. Department of Health and Human Services. *Rural Health in the People's Republic of China*. National Institutes of Health Publication No. 81-2124. Washington, D.C., 1980.

U.S. Department of Health, Education and Welfare, Public Health Service, Health Resources Administration. *Health Services Systems in the European Economic Community*. Seminar proceedings published in cooperation with the American College of Hospital Administrators. DHE Publication No. (HRA) 76-638. Washington, D.C., 1976.

van der Sprenkel, Sybille. *Legal Institutions in Manchu China*. Cambridge, Mass.: Harvard University Press, 1962.

Wegman, Myron E.; Lin, Tsung-yi; and Pucell, Elizabeth, eds. *Public*

Health in the People's Republic of China. New York: Josiah Macy, Jr., Foundation, 1973.

Wei, Min. "1979: More Than Seven Million People Employed." *Beijing Review* 23, no. 6 (11 February 1980):13–23.

Wen, C. P., and Hays, C. W. "Medical Education in China in the Postcultural Revolution Era." *New England Journal of Medicine* 292 (1975):998–1005.

White, Lynn T. *Careers in Shanghai*. Berkeley: University of California Press, 1978.

Whyte, Martin K. *Small Groups and Political Rituals in China*. Berkeley: University of California Press, 1974.

Whyte, Martin K., and Parish, William L. *Urban Life in Contemporary China*. Chicago: University of Chicago Press, 1983.

Wu, J. "The Future of Postgraduate Medical Education and Training in China." In *Medical Education in Asia: A Symposium*. New York: China Medical Board of New York, 1981.

Wu, Lien-te. *Plague Fighter: The Autobiography of a Modern Chinese Physician*. Cambridge: Heffer, 1959.

Xing, Yixun. "*Power Versus Law*, a Play in Four Acts." Translated in *Chinese Literature* 6 (June 1980):31–91.

Yang, Hsiao. *The Making of a Peasant Doctor*. Beijing: Foreign Language Press, 1976.

Zhongguo Baike Nianjian 1980 [1980 Chinese yearbook]. Beijing: Zhongguo Baike Nianjian Publishing House, 1980.

Zhou, Yiying. "The Economy." *China Reconstructs*, December 1980, 9.

Index